My Journey with Prostate Cancer of Gleason Score 8:

From Diagnosis To Remission

**Tran Van Thuong,
Professor of Mathematics**

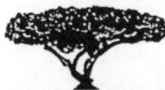

BANYAN · TREE · PRESS

BANYAN TREE PRESS

My Journey with Prostate Cancer of Gleason Score 8: From Diagnosis To Remission

ISBN: 978-1-936449-96-5

Design & Layout: Ronda Taylor, www.rondataylor.com

The following articles are Excerpted with permission from *HealthyLivinG* Magazine (HealthyLivinGMagazine.us):

"If you are undergoing chemotherapy or radiotherapy, you need to know about RNA-fragments"

"The Columbia Connection"

"How One Man's Courage is Helping Cancer Patients Across America"

"Golden Leaf Ginkgo Extract for Radiation Protection and Skin Fibrosis"

"Prostabel Reduces Men's PSA Counts" Source: *HealthyLivinG*

"Prostabel – Men's Serious Prostate Health Support" Source: *HealthyLivinG*

"High PSA, Negative Biopsy, Now What?"

The following is reprinted with permission of the publisher:

"A Story Told by an ARVN Soldier: The Need for a Formulation of a Just Cause for the ARVN"

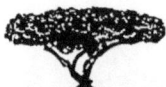

BANYAN · TREE · PRESS
Banyan Tree Press

Acknowledgments

Regarding Sylvie Beljanski, the daughter of Mirko Beljanski, PhD: She has continued to produce at least two famous products discovered by Dr. Beljanski - the Prostabel and Ginkgo V dietary supplements - that saved my life. Moreover, she also sent many documents to me that helped me learn the theory of prostate cancer deeply, and this helped me beat my cancer. To Dr. Beljanski and his daughter, I express my highest gratitude.

I thank urologist Dr. Michael Cookson, and his colleagues at the Stephenson Cancer Center Urology Department for giving me much professional and honest advice for my situation - 75 years old with prostate cancer of Gleason score 8. They educated me about Lupron hormone therapy: it could never cure my terminal prostate cancer, but would instead simply delay my death. As a matter of fact, I have had a lot of side-effects from my Lupron injection on January 22, 2016. Therefore, I decided to quit Lupron hormone therapy on April 22, 2016. At that date, Lupron therapy ceased to be effective because the injection is only effective for three months.

Thank you to Dr. Gregory Jia at Mercy Clinic Urology, Dr. Osamu Ukimura at Keck School of Medicine of USC, and Dr. Thomas Daniels at Mayo Clinic Arizona for encouraging me to take hormone therapy - one part of a feasible solution for my case.

Thank you to Dr. Larry McDade, naturopathic doctor, who reviewed my list of dietary and natural supplements.

Also, I must be grateful To Dr. Mudassir Nawaz, my family doctor, who first expressed concern for my PSA, and advised me to see a urologist as soon as possible.

Sixth, during my journey of searching for a decent publishing company, I have been lucky to meet two editors, Dr. Patricia Ross and Mr. George Gluchowski. Thank God for giving me a chance to learn from them. Their treatment of my book not only touched my heart, but also encouraged me to learn new aspects of book publication.

Seventh, I thank my two best faithful friends to me, Mr. Tran Trung Ginh and Mr. Nguyen Van Tin. In particular, Mr. Tran Trung Ginh has donated his time and computer expertise, and spent many hours editing the book. Moreover, Mr. Ginh did all this under the pressures of working a full work week and babysitting his three granddaughters.

Finally, I cannot forget my soul-mate who takes care of me in my old age, from reminding me to take my medicine to emotional support. Second, my dear son, Scott Van Thuong, who has spent a lot of time helping me with technology while he has been busy teaching and researching mathematics as a university professor.

Contents

Disclaimer

The author and/or publisher under no circumstance can guarantee that any information in this book is absolutely true.

The author and/or publisher is not a professional in any medical field. I, the author, am writing from the perspective of a soldier of the ARVN (Army of the Republic of Vietnam), who spent 15 years in the jungle, fighting side by side with American soldiers, with whom I shared the risks of combat with, as well as the increased risk of prostate cancer from the use of Agent Orange.

The author confirms that the information in this book is absolutely not medical advice for readers and prostate cancer patients. Readers and cancer patients must consult their respective medical doctors and healthcare professionals for medical advice. My lab results only apply to my particular case at a certain period of time.

Please, disavow all responsibility by the author, or/and the publisher, and/or consultants, and/or editorial content, and/or cited organizations, and/or product suppliers, and/or diagnostic and/or anything relating to my unprofessional content in this book.

Preface

There are many reasons for me to write this book. The first is to share my journey on the battlefield with prostate cancer with hope of helping others. The second is to pay respect to my comrades who share the same risk of cancer, and those who are dealing with the mental and physical pain caused by this disease. Third, it gives me great personal satisfaction to share my personal journey with a humanitarian purpose. Fourth, I am a professional educator of mathematics who has spent more than two decades in U.S. universities. Therefore, I feel it is my obligation to report my personal experience in battling a Gleason score 8 (high risk) prostate cancer.

I was a professional combat soldier of the ARVN in the Viet Nam War from the early 60's to the 70's. When I completed my military career, I had attained the rank of Lt. Colonel. There was no concept of "tour of duty" for me - I was in the jungle continuously. I was exposed to Agent Orange and radiation in the battlefield. Thanks to God, I have survived to today, I already conquered the battle against my heart condition, and I will continue to win my current battle against prostate cancer.

I spent over 10 years fighting side by side with my soldiers and my American comrades. Over time, I have witnessed many of them succumb to prostate cancer, and other cancers related to Agent Orange. It's so sad to see that they conquered many dangerous battlefields only to die of prostate cancer. In fact, there is recent scientific evidence of the link between Agent Orange and cancer. A 2013 study at the Portland VA Medical Center and

Oregon Health and Science University showed that veterans exposed to Agent Orange had not only a higher risk of prostate cancer, but are also more likely to have aggressive prostate cancer. See more at http://www.publichealth. va.gov/exposures/agentorange/conditions/prostate_cancer.asp

Dear my comrade,

I wrote this book for you and I wish all of us to stand up to fight the battle against prostate cancer together with the assistance of our urologists, oncologists, pharmaceutical companies, natural and dietary supplement companies, modern technology, many books by both patients and professionals on the subject of prostate cancer... We have a vast amount of resources and information to defeat prostate cancer today, and we learn more and more as time goes on.

1

My Journey From Military Life In Vietnam To America

I graduated from the Vietnamese Military Academy at DaLat, Vietnam in 1963 with the 17th class. I spent most of my early life in the jungles of Viet Nam engaging in combat in areas such as the Viet Cong D sanctuary and the Iron Triangle sanctuary, as well as the campaign in Cambodia. In 2004, I wrote an article on the battle of Snoul in Cambodia from my experience as battalion commander of the 1st battalion of the 8th regiment, of the fifth division of the ARVN. One of the primary reasons I wrote this was to honor the combatants who participated, as well as render justice to heroes who have been left out of ARVN military history. You can read it (in English) at http://www.generalhieu.com/snoulthuong-2.htm. Also see http://www.patriotfiles.com/archive/generalhieu/chinhnghia_arvn-2.htm.

In June 1974, I was invited, along with three other ARVN colonels to attend the U.S. Army Command and General Staff College at Fort Leavenworth, Kansas for one year of training. Thank God I had this great opportunity! I was able to expand my knowledge of military tactics and strategy at the division, corps, and national level. Moreover, many of my American classmates, such as 4 star General Wesley Clark, went on to hold high positions in the US Military and Government. I was very fortunate to be in the United States when Saigon fell in 1975. By the end of my military career, I was awarded several valor awards, including a Bronze Star (http://www.vietnamwarhonors.com/index.php?page=directory&rec=13693). But in 1975, I became a Vietnamese refugee in the United States. Thanks to God, my sponsor owned his own bank with many branches. He assigned me to be a trainee to replace the manager of one branch of his bank.

Of course, I really appreciated to have this opportunity to make a new life in America. Unfortunately, I felt bored without a challenge. So, I continued to work during the daytime, and at the same time I studied mathematics at Washburn University in Topeka, KS. As a math major, my mind was challenged everyday with difficult concepts. Thanks to the many scholarships offered by Washburn, I was eventually able to attend school full time. Thanks to the encouragement of the faculty, as well as their allowing me to test out of many classes through "credit by examination," I graduated in summer of 1977.

Then in fall of 1977, I started as a math graduate student at the University of Kansas, with the hopes of earning a PhD. I began teaching a year later in 1978 as a teaching assistant. While the title technically was "assistant," I never was an "assistant!" After a brief teaching demonstration to the faculty, I was always allowed to teach my own classes. It was difficult to teach mathematics in a language other than my mother tongue. Nevertheless, I was one of the two finalists for a teaching award in the mathematics department. I also found that the leadership skills that I had developed in my military service were applicable to the classroom. My progression through the Ph.D. program was very rapid, and I was close to finishing my research in an area of mathematics called lattice theory. However, I was interested in an area of mathematics called topology, and I made the difficult decision to transfer to the University of Utah, which at the time had a very strong topology program. So, in 1980, I said goodbye to Lawrence and moved to Salt Lake City to begin a new PhD. program. I continued teaching as a "Graduate Teaching Fellow" at Utah, and in 1986 I completed my Ph.D. in geometric topology.

Of course, what is a Ph.D. in abstract math without a job? I know many Ph.D.s in abstract math are worried about finding a job. However, I was very lucky again to find a job at the University of Minnesota – Duluth. I had a few happy years there, but I eventually took a job at Missouri Southern State University. I taught there for about 20 years before I retired in 2009.

2

My Journey As A Pro Se Representative In A Civil Rights Lawsuit And Its Consequences For My Health

I had always been in excellent health until 2004, when I turned 64. In that year, I developed a heart condition (high blood pressure and arrhythmia). Here is why I believe that I developed this condition. In 2001, I was the plaintiff in a civil rights lawsuit regarding race discrimination against my son, who was then in middle school. The defendant was a local school district, and the complaint involved school administrators ranging from the district superintendent down to a middle school principle and his assistant. The problem was that my lawyer just wanted to get money from the district. We were offered a settlement, but I chose to turn it down. My son and I were not after money; we just wanted to see the school district take responsibility and for justice to be served.

As a result of this disagreement with my lawyer, in 2003, I decided to represent my son without a lawyer, that is, *Pro se*, in the lawsuit. Because civil law was a completely new field to me, I woke up at 1 AM every morning, every day, to learn about American civil rights law. Of course, the organization I was suing had hired an excellent law firm, so it was very stressful to learn enough civil rights law to match and exceed their knowledge. This was all in addition to the teaching and research that I had to do as a professor—I did not take any time off from my job.

In the end, the lawsuit did not go to court. However, my son and I felt completely satisfied. The defendants ended up demoted to lower positions or even left the school district. In any case, at least they still had a job so they could take care of their families. In general, I believe that we must have compassion for fellow human beings when solving any problem. Before 1974, I always treated my soldiers, civilians, and captured enemies with compassion. Perhaps this is why my soldiers protected me during combat, and why I received valuable intelligence from civilians and prisoners on the enemy. It helped me survive.

While I considered the end result of the lawsuit a success, an unfortunate consequence of my grueling work routine was that I developed a heart condition (high blood pressure and arrhythmia) due to the extreme stress. This resulted in many trips to the hospital and emergency room – more than about ten times in one month! You can read some documentation below. There are over 150 pages of medical records related to this – here I only attach five pages at the end of this chapter.

In 2004, some doctors in Joplin, where I was then living, advised me to get a pacemaker inside my body, to help control my heart. I refused this rather invasive procedure, and instead tried a healthier diet, exercised seven days a week, and I found several Indian Ayurvedic herbal medicines for high blood pressure. I did not even take any of the conventional high blood pressure medications that my doctors prescribed to me. So my doctors were very surprised when they saw that I completely healed my high blood pressure and arrhythmia through natural remedies.

In addition, around 2004, I developed benign prostatic hyperplasia (BPH), which resulted in an excessive amount of nocturnal urination (http://www.urologyhealth.org/urologic-conditions/benign-prostatic-hyperplasia-d%28bph%29), and also prostatitis (http://www.mayoclinic.org/diseases-conditions/prostatitis/basics/definition/con-20020916). I suffered with this for many years, the symptoms coming and going, and often times would even experience pain when attempting to urinate. Finally, in 2009, the year that I retired, I decided to take action. I was encouraged by my success in treating my high blood pressure through natural means. By taking the Ayurstate natural supplement (traditional Indian medicine, see http://www.ayurstatedirect.com), I was able to completely eliminate my symptoms from 2009 to 2014.

In 2015, I was diagnosed with prostate cancer. Looking back at my past from 1963 until present, I just formed a theory about my prostate cancer. From 1963 until 1972, I was fighting in the jungle against the enemy, and was therefore exposed to Agent Orange 24 hours a day. Agent Orange was a herbicide used by the US Military in Vietnam to kill densely populated vegetation, so as to expose enemy positions and supply lines. It is named "Agent Orange" because of the orange striped drums used to transport and store it. Nearly 20 million gallons of it were dumped across Vietnam over the course of the war. Even my American comrades, who may have been exposed "only" for a few months to a couple of years, deserve to get assistance from our U.S. government:

(see http://www.publichealth.va.gov/PUBLICHEALTH/exposures/agentorange/benefits/index.asp)

The U.S government attests that Agent Orange is linked to many different forms of cancer, including lymphoma, soft tissue sarcoma, and lung cancer, in addition to prostate cancer. Moreover, it is also linked to birth defects in the children of those exposed. Please see more details provided by the American Cancer Society at:

http://www.cancer.org/cancer/cancercauses/othercarcinogens/intheworkplace/agent-orange-and-cancer.

In my particular case, heart disease and prostate cancer have had a significant impact on my life. Who knows how many of the about 2.6 million US veterans have, or will, develop health problems due to Agent Orange? Moreover, how many Vietnamese veterans and citizens of Vietnam have, or will, develop health problems due to Agent Orange? Many veterans who file lawsuits against the companies that produced Agent Orange were not successful.

http://www.veteranshealth.org/Vietnam/AO.html

http://www.vietnow.com/va-claims-agent-orange/

http://www.agentorangerecord.com/information/the_quest_for_additional_relief/

For deeper information on Agent Orange, please, read this reference: https://en.wikipedia.org/wiki/Agent_Orange

As for myself, my heart problem and prostate cancer with Gleason score 8 is empirical evidence of the impact Agent Orange has had on my health. Moreover, there are thousands of my American and Vietnamese comrades with different types of cancer nowadays. Perhaps we will need many high powered lawyers to win a lawsuit someday in the future.

My prostate cancer is the most difficult battlefield that I have ever fought in my life. The rest of the book is devoted to this battlefield.

HISTORY & PHYSICAL AND DISCHARGE SUMMARY

FREEMAN HEALTH SYSTEM

NAME: THUONG,TRAN V   CHART #:   ADMITTED: 03/12/04

DOCTOR: Nicholas,W John MD   DISCHARGED:
===

DIAGNOSIS: 1) Atrial flutter with a rapid ventricular response. This appears
                  to be new onset atrial flutter.
               2) Newly recognized hypertension this week.

DISCHARGE MEDICATIONS: Cardizem CD 240 q d, Dyazide 1 q d.

FOLLOW UP: The patient will follow-up in the next two to three days with Dr.
Dougherty and myself.   ,

CLINICAL RESUME AND HOSPITAL COURSE: Tran Thuong is a 63 year old Vietnamese
gentleman who was admitted through the Emergency Room early this morning with
hypertension and palpitations. Earlier this week he had been diagnosed with new
onset hypertension. He was begun initially on Clonidine and subsequently on
Zestril. With both medications he believes that he had severe reactions. He has
been insomnic for the past three days. He attributes this to the medications. He
had a normal stress echocardiogram with good exercise tolerance.

The patient insisted that he has always been in good health and he feels something
is very wrong of recent. He is taking a bee pollen/honey which he purchases at
Suzanne's. It is called Royal Jelly. He has taken this extensively in the past
but apparently last week when he took it he developed some reactions which he
believes began a cascade of problems, particularly this high blood pressure. He
has had some headaches and had a negative CT scan last week.

ALLERGIES: None known.

MEDICATIONS: None until recently and only recently the patient has been on the
Zestril and Clonidine.

PAST MEDICAL HISTORY: Noncontributory.

PAST SURGICAL HISTORY: None.

SOCIAL HISTORY: The patient is a math professor at MSSU. He does not smoke or
drink.

FAMILY HISTORY: Negative for early coronary artery disease.

REVIEW OF SYSTEMS: The patient has a very active lifestyle. He has not had
paroxysmal nocturnal dyspnea, orthopnea, syncope or predictable exertional chest
discomfort. Other review of systems are noncontributory.

FINAL DIAGNOSIS: 1) ATRIAL FLUTTER WHICH RESOLVED ON A CARDIZEM DRIP EARLY THIS
                        MORNING.
                     2) NEWLY DIAGNOSED HYPERTENSION.

===
                 HISTORY & PHYSICAL AND DISCHARGE SUMMARY
PRINTED 03/12/04
         0959

Page 1 of 2

9

3

The Beginning Of My Journey With Prostate Cancer

Because I was able to eliminate my symptoms of BPH from 2009 to 2014, and my last PSA test (prostate-specific antigen) in 2009 was well under 4.0 ng/mL, I was completely confident in my health and decided to forgo PSA testing during those years. Nevertheless, in October of 2015, my intuition told me that I ought to get a PSA test. At that time, I didn't have any symptoms of prostate enlargement, and I was able to urinate just fine. Moreover, I was able to sleep through the night, only using the bathroom a couple of times. Unfortunately, I received the results of my PSA test on October 22, 2015, and I was shocked to see that my PSA was high at 15.9 ng/mL. My family doctor, Dr. Mudassir Nawaz immediately advised me to see a urologist. When I hesitated, he asked for my wife and son's contact information, so that they could convince me to see a urologist. Eventually, I knew that something had to be done, and I finally decided to see a urologist, Dr. Edward Dakil.

Upon reviewing my medical records, my urologist advised me to get a prostate biopsy right away. Having done some research on the potential side effects, I wasn't so enthusiastic for this course of action. Nevertheless, I was okay with the prospect of an MRI of my pelvic region and prostate, as it is a non-invasive test. On October 26, 2015, I received the report from the radiologist, Dr. Guatam Dehadrai.

In the report, the radiologist found a 2.8 cm lesion on my prostate, which was "suspicious." It was also alarming that he found a suspicious area on my right pubic bone, a possible signal that cancer had spread there from my prostate. But even with this news, I still hesitated to do the prostate biopsy. After all, I felt completely healthy. Why not just try a "watch and wait" approach? So, I wanted to try to find a second opinion.

Norman Regional Health System

| MOORE MEDICAL CENTER | HEALTHPLEX MEDICAL CENTER
DX REPORT
MRI PELVIS W/O CONTRAST | NORMAN REGIONAL HOSPITAL |

Patient Name: THUONG,TRAN V	Unit #:	Acct #:
DOB:	Age: 75	Sex: M
Ordering MD: S Edward Dakil, MD	Order #: 1026-0020	Order Date: 10/26/15
Room:	Location: HRAD	Report #:1026-0466
Procedure Dt/Time: 10/26/15 1334	Accession#	

Signed

Clinical history: Prostate enlargement.

Comparison: None.

Findings: Diffuse enlargement prostate producing stenosis and leftward deviation of urethra and mass effect on bladder base. Approximately 2.8 cm peripheral lesion demonstrating restricted diffusion with T1 low and T2 high signal within left posterolateral aspect of prostate gland, highly suspicious for neoplasm. Lesion appears to remain superior to the urogenital diaphragm. Urinary bladder normal in size. Ill-defined bone marrow T1 low signal and T2 high signal within right superior pubic ramus, demonstrating restricted diffusion, highly suspicious for a neoplastic process such as metastatic disease. No gross pelvic adenopathy. No free fluid within pelvis.

Impression: Focus of restricted diffusion left posterolateral peripheral aspect of prostate gland, highly suspicious for neoplasm. Abnormal bone marrow signal within right superior pubic ramus, suspicious for metastatic disease. Diffuse enlargement prostate.

CC: Dakil,S Edward, MD
Nawaz,Mudassir, MD

Transcribed By: Gautam Dehadrai
Transcribed Time: 10/26/15 1427

Dictated by: Dehadrai,Gautam, MD
Dictated Date/Time: 10/26/15 1427

Signed by: Dehadrai,Gautam, MD
Signed by Date/Time: 10/26/15 1507
Co Signed by:
Co Signed by Time:
Co Signed Date:

4

The Search For A Second Opinion, My Prostate Biopsy, Its Consequences

First, I consulted with Dr. Michael Cookson, Chairman and Professor of Urology at OU Medical Center, about Dr. Dehadrai's evaluation of my pelvis MRI. He suggested a prostate cancer biopsy. Second, on November 17, 2015, I traveled to Los Angeles for a consultation with Dr. Osamu Ukimura at the medical school of the University of Southern California. I was not too enthused with the idea of a prostate biopsy, and I wanted to find an alternate approach. But after Dr. Ukimura saw the result of the MRI, he also told me that I needed a prostate biopsy as soon as possible. A few days later, I traveled to Dallas for a consultation with Dr. Claus Roehrburn at UT Southwestern Medical Center. He suggested that I should have my prostate removed immediately. The side effects of this scared me even more than getting a biopsy – one of my concerns was that I would be forced to wear a urinary catheter my entire life. I was also seventy-five years old, and I did not know if I could make it through the surgery without serious complications.

Having consulted many experienced and prestigious urologists, my mind was made up: I had to get to a biopsy. So on December 17, 2015, I had my biopsy at Mercy Hospital in Oklahoma City with Dr. Gregory Jia.

I chose to have this urologist do the biopsy for two reasons: first, I felt very comfortable with him, second, he used the ultrasound to guide the needle probe. Apparently, not all urologists use ultrasound during prostate biopsies. I went under full anesthesia, and upon waking up found myself extremely nauseous (which I think was due to the anesthesia), and had severe vomiting all through the car ride back home.

Just two days later on December 19, 2015, I woke up to an alarming amount of blood in my urine. While I knew a prostate biopsy would result in blood, I felt the amount was excessive. So I was rushed to the emergency room at Norman Regional Hospital because of heavy bleeding. Apparently, there was not much the doctor could do to stop the bleeding, but my blood work came back normal, so I had not lost a dangerous amount of blood. Then the next day on December 20, I returned to the emergence room again because of blood in my stool. Thankfully, the ER doctor did not find a dangerous amount of blood in my stool, and he also used an ultrasound to search for any internal bleeding, which thankfully again none was found. After a few more days, the bleeding stopped.

On December 23, 2015, I returned to Mercy Hospital to get the results of my prostate biopsy from Dr. Jia. Of the six areas they biopsied on my prostate, one was benign, one had a Gleason score of 7, and the remaining four had a Gleason score of 8. The Gleason score is a number from 2 to 10 which represents a rough estimate of how aggressive the cancer is. The higher the Gleason score, the more aggressive the cancer. the At this point, Dr. Jia suggested I get a chest X-ray, as well as a bone scan to verify that the cancer had not spread outside the prostate. A Gleason score of 8 means that the cancer has a higher risk of spreading. I was very hesitant to get the chest X-ray and bone scan; I had been exposed to so much radiation over my lifetime in the battlefield. Why should I increase my risk of secondary cancers in the future?

Nevertheless, after many doctors trying to convince me that the radiation dosage of a bone scan would not increase my risk of secondary cancer considerably, I finally elected to have my bone scan at OU Medical Center, while forgoing the chest X-ray. Supposedly, the bone scan showed a suspicious area on public bone.

Thuong, Tran   Printed 12/23/15 11:05 AM

Results   PATHOLOGY (Order 165342658)

Collection Information

Collected:	12/17/2015 9:18 AM
Collected:	12/17/2015 9:18 AM
Collected:	12/17/2015 9:18 AM
Collected:	12/17/2015 9:18 AM
Collected:	12/17/2015 9:18 AM
Collected:	12/17/2015 9:18 AM

| Specimen Type | Specimen Source |
| Tissue [117] | Prostate [432] |

Case Report

CASE REPORT

Surgical Pathology Report   Case: OS15-17526

Authorizing Provider: Jia, Gregory Y, MD   Collected:
12/17/2015 09:18 AM
Ordering Location: Mercy Outpatient   Received:
 12/17/2015 10:26 AM
                       Diagnostics Oklahoma City

Pathologist: Powers, Michelle, MD

Specimens: A) - Prostate, right base

             B) - Prostate, right mid
right mid
             C) - Prostate, right apex

             D) - Prostate, left base

             E) - Prostate, left mid

             F) - Prostate, left apex

FINAL DIAGNOSIS
A. PROSTATE, RIGHT BASE (NEEDLE BIOPSY):
-- BENIGN PROSTATIC TISSUE.

B. PROSTATE, RIGHT MID (NEEDLE BIOPSY):
-- ADENOCARCINOMA, GLEASON GRADE 4 + 4 = SCORE OF 8.
-- TUMOR PRESENT IN ONE OF TWO CORES, MEASURING 1 MM IN TOTAL LENGTH,
   COMPRISING APPROXIMATELY 3% OF THE TOTAL PROSTATIC TISSUE.

C. PROSTATE, RIGHT APEX (NEEDLE BIOPSY):
-- ADENOCARCINOMA, GLEASON GRADE 4 + 4 = SCORE OF 8.
-- TUMOR PRESENT IN ONE OF TWO CORES, MEASURING 2 MM IN TOTAL LENGTH,
   COMPRISING APPROXIMATELY 10% OF THE TOTAL PROSTATIC TISSUE.

D. PROSTATE, LEFT BASE (NEEDLE BIOPSY):
-- ADENOCARCINOMA, GLEASON GRADE 3 + 4 = SCORE OF 7.
-- TUMOR PRESENT IN TWO OF THREE CORES, MEASURING 2 MM IN TOTAL LENGTH,
   COMPRISING APPROXIMATELY 9% OF THE TOTAL PROSTATIC TISSUE.

Authorization of Releasing my Bone Scan

My name is Tran Van Thuong, _____ , and I authorize Dr. Michael S. Cookson, to release the record of Radiology OU Department Reports (NM Bone/Image whole Body which consist of a written report and a CD of the image) to:

Mayo Clinic
Please, fax to:
Debbie Thoumsin
Radiation Oncology
Fax # : 480-342-3972
Phone: 480-342-1262
Address: Radiation Oncology
5777 E Mayo Blvd, Phoenix, AZ 85054

Tran Van Thuong

Jan 7, 2016

5

My Strategic Decision Of Selecting A Course Of Treatment

Having received the result of my bone scan, I consulted with Dr. Cookson at OU Cancer Center, as well as his team of urologists. All three uniformly suggested Lupron hormone therapy. Dr. Jia also had the same idea. After sending the result of my bone scan to Mayo Clinic in Phoenix, AZ, I traveled there on January 20, 2016 to see Dr. Thomas Daniels, and even he had the same idea. At this point, all the doctors considered the cancer "metastatic," that is, the cancer had spread to the bone, according to the bone scan. Therefore, hormone therapy was the standard treatment plan that conventional medicine prescribed.

Using the Internet, I investigated and researched what supplements could reduce oxidative stress and inflammatory stress (also see Chapter 7). Readers should know that information on the Internet is not a reliable source of medical information. Readers should do their own research and take responsibility for evaluating the information that they find before they select their holistic supplements for treatment of prostate cancer.

NOTE: The author confirms that the information in this book does not constitute medical advice for readers and prostate cancer patients. Readers and cancer patients must consult their medical doctors and their health care professionals if seeking medical advice. Again, all of my results and lab work only apply to my specific case at that period of time.

Here is what I found from the Internet. Please, read the information and think it over.

1. Pomi-T contains pomegranate, green tea, broccoli, and turmeric. A study of 203 men with localized prostate cancer at Bedford Hospital and Addenbrooke's Hospital in the United Kingdom showed a statistically significant effect on slowing down increase of PSA. You can read more at:
http://www.pomi-t.com/asco-pomi-t-study-summary/
https://www.21co.com/lasvegas/news/prostate-cancer-may-be-controlled-pomi-t-supplement
http://www.pomi-t.com/faq-pomi-t/
http://prostatecanceruk.org/about-us/news-and-views/2013/6/superfoods

2. Supercritical Prostate 5LX. This supplement contains various phytonutrients (from plants) such as nettle, saw palmetto. It also contains selenium, rosemary, and green tea. You can read more at: https://www.newchapter.com/targeted-herbal-formulas/prostate-5lx

3. Turkey Tail Mushroom for Immune System. Turkey Tail Mushroom has been used in Asia for many years for its medicinal benefits. Furthermore, recently there has been scientific evidence to its effectiveness. For example, a study at the Queensland University of Technology demonstrated that a compound (polysaccharopeptide) in the mushroom was effective in targeting prostate cancer stem cells and suppressed tumor formation in mice. Moreover, the FDA recently approved a clinical trial at Bastyr Integrative Oncology Research Center around 2012. You can read more at:
https://www.sciencedaily.com/releases/2011/05/110523091539.htm
http://www.bastyr.edu/news/general-news/2012/11/fda-approves-bastyr-turkey-tail-trial-cancer-patients
http://depts.washington.edu/integonc/clinicians/act/mushroom_extracts.shtml
http://www.drugs.com/npp/turkey-tail.html
http://www.wildernesscollege.com/turkey-tail-mushrooms.html
https://www.mskcc.org/cancer-care/integrative-medicine/herbs/coriolus-versi-color

4. Prostate Revive. Prostate Revive contains 15 ingredients that support prostate health, including saw palmetto and pomegranate extract. After age forty, a man's body converts testosterone in to the compound DHT (dihydrotestosterone). DHT is thought to be one of the reasons the prostate gland gets bigger as a man ages. Prostate Revive was formulated to help block the conversion of testosterone to DHT and therefore prevent inflammation of the prostate. You can read more at: http://www.medixselect.com/product/PR_Bundle/products http://buyerreview.com/medix-select-prostate-revive-supplement-reviews/ http://www.manrelated.com/prostate-revive

5. Prostabel is a product developed by Dr. Mirko Beljanski, specifically for the prostate, as the name implies. It contains Pao Pereira extract and powdered Rauwolfia vomitoria extract. Dr. Aaron Katz, a urologist and founder of Columbia University Center for Holistic Oncology, showed that Prostabel can significantly lower a man's PSA in twelve months, as well as improve urinary function. You can read more at the following link, and in the two articles below. You can also find several scientific articles in the appendix detailing the anti-cancer effects of Pao Pereira and Rauwolfia vomitoria. https://www.beljanskiproducts.com/products/prostabel/

6. Ginkgo V. This supplement was developed by Dr. Beljanski. It consists of powdered golden leaf ginkgo extract. It works at the cellular level and prevents cells from being damaged by rogue enzymes. Information about the supplement can be found at: https://www.beljanskiproducts.com/products/gingko-v/ http://www.naturalhealthconsult.com/all-products/669.html http://natural-remedies.healthgrove.com/compare/43-54/Ginkgo-vs-Iron Moreover, a 2003 article of DeFeudis, Papadopoulos, and Drieu (http://www.ncbi.nlm.nih.gov/pubmed/12914542) appearing in the Journal of Fundamental & Clinical Pharmacology supports the anti-cancer properties of ginkgo. (The abstract can be found at the given link.)

7. GeniKinoko. This supplement contains GCP (genistein combined polysaccharide), a byproduct produced by fermentation of soybean isoflavone extracts with basidiomycetes mushrooms.
   http://www.betterhealthinternational.com/productDetails.asp?prodID=QOL101

8. Swanson Ultra Max-Strength Graminex Flower Pollen Extract. This supplement contains flower pollen extracts that enhance and maintain prostate and urinary health. These extracts have been in use in Europe and Asia for more than thirty years.
   http://www.swansonvitamins.com/swanson-ultra-max-strength-graminex-flower-pollen-ext-500-mg-60

9. Quality of Life Labs Kinoko Gold. 1-800-678-8989 or 1-800-226-2370. This supplement contains Active Hexose Correlated Compound (AHCC), an extract from several species of mushrooms. AHCC improves immune system response, so that the body can destroy cancer cells more easily.

10. Finally, perhaps a special kind of "medicine" without any physical manifestation may give cancer patients the power to destroy all forms of cancer. This medicine that I am referring to is love and compassion for others. Thanks to Dr. David Hawkins, Ph.D., a philosopher, scientist, and a great mathematician, for this wonderful idea.
    https://en.wikipedia.org/wiki/David_Hawkins_%28philosopher%29
    https://dancewithtruth.wordpress.com/dr-david-hawkins-quotes/

I would like to share my personal experience with readers. I consistently fought against the enemy (prostate cancer) from the day I was diagnosed until I completely defeated the cancer. I have never been angry, but I have always been compassionate with patients like myself, as well as loving poor people. Therefore, I have had neither internal nor external enemies.

I have many friends with prostate cancer. Most of them have the same personal character as myself, and I often meet them at the doctor's office for cancer treatment. Some other people have a hostile personality, and it was rare to meet them, perhaps they gave up treatment? I was lucky to know about David Hawkins, Ph.D., who gave me encouragement and hope.

In addition to the above supplements, a clean and healthy lifestyle has been very important to conquering my prostate cancer. Having a peaceful mind and exercising everyday strengthened my immune system to fight cancer.

....

DIET

Diet is a major lifestyle component, and I wanted to give my body all the fuel it needed to defeat cancer. The search for my personal anti-cancer diet began with the question: "What foods cause cancerous cells to grow and develop in our bodies?" In other words, what foods do cancerous cells like to eat so that they multiply? By eliminating such foods from my diet, I planned to starve the cancer cells to their death.

Healthy, non-cancerous cells in our body are genetically programmed to die on their own. This process is known as apoptosis (from the Greek word for "falling off"). As old cells die off, they are replaced with new, healthy cells, and this cycle of life allows the body to continue to live with good health. The problem with cancerous cells is that they lack the genetic programming for apoptosis. That is, as long as they are provided with the appropriate nutrients, they will continue to multiply and never commit suicide.

Based on my research, I came up with a theory: by eating carcinogen-free foods that reduce oxidative stress and inflammation, this would fuel the immune system, while depriving cancer cells of the food they need to grow. That is, I planned to only eat foods that cancer didn't want to eat! By starving the cancer cells of the carcinogenic food that they need, perhaps we can induce them to begin the process of apoptosis, thus killing themselves off.

Therefore, most of my diet consists purely of organic fruits, vegetables, grains, and legumes. I get my all of my animal protein from wild caught seafood and organic eggs. The more unprocessed the food, the better. I avoid all other forms of meat, dairy, refined sugars, and processed foods. Furthermore, a healthy diet begins with a pure water supply. To avoid carcinogens potentially lurking in tap water, I always drink and cook with reverse-osmosis filtered water.

Why do I believe that my empirical theory is true? The answer is provided by observing my own recovery from prostate cancer. Before discovering my own diet, I felt pain around my pelvic bone. I had painful urination, and it was hard to have regular bowel movements. However, now I feel urination is so easy, and I am never constipated. After one month on my new diet, something surprised me. One morning, after a bowel movement, my stool had a terrible odor. I felt a release inside my body and the pain in my pelvic bone decreased over the next week. For one week I had smelly bowel movements, and then it stopped. I know that the cancer cells died off—they may have been starved to death.

However, how should I prove that my empirical theory is true using the scientific method? That is an open and challenging question. Perhaps a biologist can study the chemical properties of the foods in my diet, and then come up with his or her theory. Nevertheless, the diet that worked for me may not work for everyone. Indeed, I was the only subject studied. Therefore, a biologist would need to conduct a randomized experiment with a very large sample size of people, categorized into many different groups. Finally, the biologist would use mathematical probability and statistics to summarize the results for the sample of people, as well as generalize the results from the sample to the general population.

For the rest of Chapter 5, I will list in detail the various kinds of anti-cancer foods, as well as recipes that I use. Here is how I eat everyday:

BREAKFAST:

I start my day in the morning with a six ounce cup of unsweetened homemade soy yogurt. Here is how I make it. I have a simple yogurt maker which will make seven servings, so you should only have to make yogurt once a week with this yogurt maker. Follow the instructions that come with your yogurt maker. With my yogurt maker, I prefer to use organic soy milk (unsweetened). For every forty-eight ounces of soy milk, I use six ounces of unsweetened coconut milk yogurt as a culture starter. Use whatever brand you prefer, but I would just suggest all ingredients to be unsweetened, so as to reduce your refined sugar consumption.

I also eat a bowl of organic oatmeal or organic oat bran. Finally, I drink a six-ounce cup of shake. In a blender, I mix half an organic small apple, half an organic small avocado, and some organic unsweetened soymilk.

LUNCH:

At lunch, I eat a medley of organic fruits and vegetables: cauliflower, broccoli, daikon, carrots, half an avocado, tomatoes, cucumbers, and red and green bell peppers.

I also prepare a bowl of cooked greens, consisting of kale and mustard, turnip, or collard greens. Kale is rather easy to find organic, but organic varieties of the rest can be difficult to find. I simply place the carefully washed greens in a large pan, add a couple cups of water, and cook it on low to medium heat until they are tender. I season it with sea salt, and also tabasco sauce. Sometimes I also add a hot pepper (Anaheim, Jalapeno, or Habanero, from mildest to hotter). There is some scientific evidence that capsaicin, the chemical that makes the pepper hot, may help against prostate cancer.

Then I cook two ounces of organic quinoa, a grain that is very high in protein. My dessert consists of organic fruit, such as blueberries, blackberries, apples, or peaches (depending on the season, and only one type per day).

SATURDAY: JUICE DETOX

Saturday is a special day of the week. I add one more item to my lunch: a 16 oz drink made by juicing organic celery, cucumbers, (red) kale, beets, carrots, a quarter of a lemon, and half an apple.

DINNER:

Dinner changes every day, and Saturday's dinner rotates every week. One item that is a constant at every dinner is fresh organic vegetables. I choose from romaine lettuce, red leaf romaine lettuce, iceberg lettuce, asparagus, radishes, green onion, watercress, alfalfa sprouts, parsley, and cilantro. Generally, I just pick three for dinner.

On Monday, I eat organic spaghetti with organic spaghetti squash and organic spaghetti sauce.

On Tuesday, I eat canned, wild caught, sardines with organic wild rice.

As for Wednesday, I eat an organic vegetarian hamburger patty and look for a brand that has the most natural ingredients. Generally, I do not eat a bun, but if I do, I choose a sprouted wheat bun. With this, I eat a guacamole salad. I cut iceberg lettuce into very small pieces, and mix this with avocado and salsa.

On Thursday, I eat organic vegetarian black bean chili. For simplicity, I use a canned brand. It comes in a can, but when you heat it with onions, yellow zucchini, and cilantro, it tastes just like homemade chili.

As for Friday's dinner, I boil an organic free range egg, and eat it with plenty of organic wild rice and organic vegetables.

I have three different options for dinner on Saturday. Option one is a vegetarian taco dinner, again, with all organic ingredients (even the blue corn taco shell). The filling of the taco is made from organic refried black beans, tomatoes, green onions, lettuce, cilantro, and guacamole.

The second option on Saturday is a very simple no-cheese pizza. I use a pre-made organic whole wheat pizza crust. Simply top the pizza crust with organic tomato paste or sauce, and then with vegetables of your choice. After baking it, the result is a delicious and healthy pizza. I eat about one-fourth of it.

The third option on Saturday is baked wild caught Alaskan sockeye salmon, again with plenty of organic vegetables.

On Sunday, I eat a light dinner, mostly comprised of steamed vegetables (including broccoli and cauliflower) and purple potatoes (sometimes sweet and sometimes not).

After all these dinners, I have some organic fruit for dessert. Again, I believe that eating refined sugars creates an environment in our bodies that is favorable for cancers. So, I completely replace cake, cookies, and candy with organic fruit.

6

Case Studies

In this chapter, we present fifteen informative case studies which I used in formulating my strategy for battling my prostate cancer.

Case Study 1 —

An article of Reuter, et al. [Reuter] provides strong scientific evidence linking elevated levels of oxidative stress, inflammation, and cancer together. Oxidative stress is an imbalance between production of free radicals and reactive metabolites (also known as reactive oxygen species (ROS)), and elimination of these harmful compounds by means of antioxidants. The article shows that oxidative stress can activate many transcription factors, which are proteins that control gene expressions. These transcription factors can lead to the expression of over five-hundred genes, and some of these genes can result in harmful inflammation in the body. The article examines precisely how oxidative stress activates inflammatory pathways, which can result in the transformation of a normal cell to a tumor cell, survival of the tumor cell, replication of the tumor cell, and finally metastasis of the tumor cells.

Mentioned in the article is the connection between reactive oxygen species and many different diseases and cancer, in particular, to diabetes, inflammatory joint disease, Parkinson's disease, brain cancer, liver cancer, lung cancer, melanoma, leukemia, lymphoma, oral cancer, pancreatic cancer, and prostate cancer.

The authors conclude that targeting inflammation in the body can help with cancer prevention. The authors note that many natural medicines derived from "fruits, vegetables, spices, grains, and cereals" can suppress tumor formation in preclinical models, providing hope that they can do the same in patients.

Case Study 2 —

PectaSol-C Modified Citrus Pectin is another useful supplement. It is derived from the peel of citrus fruits. Its manufacturer purports that it supports healthy cell growth, normal tissue health, and healthy immune system function. PectaSol-C is a special type of pectin developed by Dr. Isaac Elizas, MD, which is specifically formulated to be easily absorbed into the bloodstream. A clinical trial demonstrated that PectaSol-C has the ability to help detoxify the body of heavy metals, and a study reported that PectaSol-C significantly decreased lead levels in children who were suffering from lead poisoning. Moreover, PectaSol-C contains polysaccharide components that researchers have shown to support Natural Killer cell activation, which are beneficial immune system cells. By interacting with galectin-3, PectaSol-C could help control inflammation levels in the body.

Most importantly for our situation, a cell model based on abnormal prostate cancer cells was actually used to develop the formula for the pectin in PectaSol-C. Moreover, several studies [Sturm, Guess] have shown that modified citrus pectin can slow the increase of PSA. You can read more at:

http://www.lifeextension.com/vitamins-supplements/item00342/pectasol-c-modified-citrus-pectin

Also, several unofficial reviews from users of PectaSol-C state that PectaSol-C helped reduce internal inflammation levels in their body. See, for example,

http://www.amazon.com/EcoNugenics-PectaSol-C-Modified-Citrus-Pectin/product-reviews/B0027VT510

Case Study 3 —

Any plan to conquer prostate cancer must have both defensive and offensive components. Readers can make their own plan after reading information from the four books listed in the references [Goldstone1], [Goldstone2], [Walker], and [Cohen]. Readers also have the option of evaluating the information in those books by consulting an ND (natural doctor), who has the same number of years of medical training as an MD.

Here is some more information on natural approaches for treating prostate cancer. By simply changing your diet, you can help your body defeat prostate cancer. For example, Lycopene, an antioxidant found in foods like tomatoes and watermelon, was found in some studies to reduce prostate cancer risk. However, the studies were not able to verify this if Lycopene was taken in supplement form. So, perhaps one should be sure to include a lot of Lycopene in their diet.

In addition, several studies have shown that Vitamin D may help defend against prostate cancer. Vitamin D can be obtained from exposure to the sun, but this can be difficult to ensure, so daily supplements can be a good way to make sure you get enough Vitamin D.

Omega-3 fatty acids are found in abundance in oily fish such as salmon and mackerel. A 2009 study considered 466 men with aggressive prostate cancer and 478 similarly aged men without prostate cancer. The study found that higher dietary intake of omega-3 fatty acids was correlated with lower risk of aggressive prostate cancer. The study hypothesized that the reduced risk was due to the ability of omega-3s to reduce inflammation. A study of 49,920 men (aged 40 to 69) published in 2008 showed that consuming green tea may also reduce your risk of prostate cancer.

Read more (along with references to the scientific articles) at:

http://altmedicine.about.com/od/cance1/a/prostate_cancer_prevention.htm

Apparently, the Cancer Treatment Center of America uses nutrition therapy in addition to conventional therapy:

http://www.cancercenter.com/treatments/nutrition-therapy/

Case Study 4 —

Daniel J. Goldstone is in 100 percent remission due to his holistic approach. You can find more information in the two books [Goldstone1, Goldstone2] listed in the references. He also updates his website at http://wwwibeatcancerholistically.com. Mr. Goldstone was hospitalized as a child due to a bleeding kidney. Going through three different doctors and two different hospitals, he learned from a young age that the medical community is still learning about the human body and does not have perfect answers. This experience gave him confidence in taking a holistic approach to curing his prostate cancer. Mr. Goldstone has also extended his anti-cancer regimen to breast, colon, and lung cancer as well [Goldstone2].

Both of his books are well-written, with documentation, to prove that his prostate cancer is in remission. He also updates his website regularly with lab results, demonstrating the continued success of his methods.

He first started on hormone therapy and radiation. Mr. Goldstone describes the rather severe side effects that hormone therapy had. However, I have not had such severe side effects. After trying these conventional treatments and suffering side effects that greatly reduced his quality of life, he decided to develop his own holistic approach to beat his cancer.

Case Study 5 —

This is the very sad case of Mr. Charlie Redd. He died with dignity after about twelve years of fighting prostate cancer. The more I read his memoir, the more I respect his patience and courage to deal with the beast of cancer. I wish that he still survived to today, so that he may have had the option of using Mr. Goldstone's holistic approach to cure himself of prostate cancer.

Mr. Redd's journey began in February of 2000, when he was diagnosed with prostate cancer at the age of 64. His initial PSA was 8.90 ng/mL, with a Gleason score of 7, and had a staging of T1c, meaning that the cancer was too small to be detected in a digital rectal exam.

Dr. John Koval, an associate of Dr. Michael Dattoli (a well-known prostate doctor in Sarasota, Florida), started Mr. Redd on Casodex on March 10, 2000. Ten days later, he received a month injection of 7.5 mg of Lupron due to the rather large size (50 grams) of his prostate and high Gleason score. A month after this, he received a three month injection of 22.5 mg of Lupron.

On November 12, 2007, Mr. Redd and his wife discovered a supplement called Prostosol online ($75 for 80 capsules, a minimum of two bottles). He was not very optimistic about this supplement, but nevertheless tried it. Prostosol was successful in reducing his PSA for many years.

Apparently though, Prostasol may increase your risk of blood clots, and Mr. Redd experienced a blood clot while on Prostasol. It is possible that

Prostasol contains either diethylstilboestrol (DES) or estradiol, which can lower PSA, but also increases the risk of blood clots. In fact, because of the risk, DES is usually prescribed with a blood thinner like Coumadin. However, other sources claim that Prostatsol contains neither DES nor estradiol, but instead a phytoestrogen, a natural ingredient. In any case, it is not clear.

Unfortunately, on April 3, 2012, Mr. Redd posted an update with the unfortunate news that the cancer had metastasized to his right hip and spine. Below is record of his PSA from 3/31/11 to 3/19/12:

  03/31/11 7.56
  04/13/11 7.65
  05/13/11 10.92
  05/26/11 10.35
  06/09/11 10.97
  07/07/11 10.60
  11/21/11 27.34
  11/29/11 28.08
  12/06/11 30.85 Lupron and Casodex started
  12/15/11 32.41
  12/21/11 41.69
  12/28/11 36.90
  01/04/12 38.90
  01/12/12 42.09
  01/18/12 47.9
  02/13/12 80.35
  02/17/12 93.00
  03/11/12 ZYTIGA (abiraterone acetate) started
  03/19/12 89.4

As these PSA measurements show, by this time, Mr. Redd was "hormone refractory," that is, the prostate cancer in his body had developed a resistance to the hormone therapy. In medical jargon, he was a man with mCRPC (metastatic castration-resistant prostate cancer). Unfortunately, he could not afford advanced conventional treatments like traveling to Sand Lake Imaging, in Orlando, to find out if the cancer had spread to his lymph nodes. He would have planned to follow this with treatment from Dr.

Datolli in Sarasota, Florida which would include DART (dynamic adaptive radiation therapy) and Samarium-153 injection (a form of radiation therapy). Instead, he tried Zytiga.

And finally, I read with tears:

> *"With great sadness I wanted to let YANA know that my wonderful sweet Charlie Redd passed away on June 4, 2013. His prostate cancer had spread to his spine and he was bedridden for 7 months. With Hospice care he was able to be at home all the time. By the Grace of God he was in very little pain. His death was very peaceful with most of the family around him. His memorial service will be at North Merritt Island Methodist Church in Merritt Island, FL on June 15, 2013, 11:00 am.*
>
> *Blessing to everyone fighting this dreadful disease.*
>
> *Take care, Charlie's wife Beverly Redd"*

You can read about Charlie Redd's story in his own words at http://www.yananow.org/display_story.php?id=162.

Case Study 6 —

George Hardy was fifty-four when he was diagnosed with prostate cancer in April of 2005. His initial PSA was very high at 182, and he had a Gleason Score of 6. His choice of conventional treatment was hormone therapy and external beam radiation.

When he was diagnosed in April of 2005, all scans initially showed that the prostate cancer was confined to the prostate and had not spread outside of it. Mr. Hardy began hormone therapy on April 26th (six 50 mg tablets of Cyproterone daily). On May 12, the Cyproterone was stopped and he began receiving Zoladex implants. On May 15, Mr. Hardy began the Jane Plant diet, which is a diet that basically excludes all dairy foods and processed foods. It is an anti-cancer diet.

Unfortunately, on May 23, 2005, an MRI showed that the cancer had spread to the left seminal vesicle. The good news was that on July 21, 2005, his PSA had fallen to 3.3. The Zoladex treatments continued into August, and on August 9, an MRI scan showed a reduction in the size of the cancerous areas. On September 21, Mr. Hardy began radiation therapy. His

PSA was now only 2.01 on September 27, but on that day he also learned that the right side of his pelvic wall was cancerous.

In October of 2005, the radiation therapy caused inflammation in the area around the prostate, restricting urine flow, and so Mr. Hardy was put on Flomax to help with urination. The good news was that on October 13, his PSA was just 0.9. He also continued on Zoladex.

In August 2006, his PSA was less than 0.1. On December of 2006, his PSA was still less than 0.1, although he reported low testosterone, which he hypothesized was causing the extreme fatigue that he was feeling. Over the next years, he used both hormone therapy and the Jane Plant diet to control his PSA levels. There also was a delicate balancing act to keep testosterone at an acceptable level so Mr. Hardy would not feel fatigued. As of his March 2016 update, his PSA was 0.41, with a decreasing trend.

So what can we learn from this? Perhaps the Jane Plant diet of avoiding dairy products and processed foods helped him beat the prostate cancer. Read about George Hardy's story in his own words at http://www.yananow.org/display_story.php?id=376.

Case Study 7 —

Dr. Jay S Cohen, author of [Cohen], is in fact a prostate cancer survivor. He used the game plan of "active surveillance protocol" to defeat his prostate cancer, which had a Gleason score of 6. Although his PSA had been high, he never adopted any conventional treatment. He survived to today to write his book, and is healthy nowadays.

Case Study 8 —

https://www.youtube.com/watch?v=BJuKm8mtATc

In this video, you can see Dr. Katz (author of [Katz]) discuss natural approaches to curing prostate cancer. He describes a study comparing outcomes of men that received no screening vs those who received active yearly PSA screening. Interestingly, studies have shown that there is little difference in prostate cancer survival rates between these two groups. The reason is that many cases do not need to be treated conventionally, but can instead be treated with an "active surveillance" approach, and in particular, an "active holistic surveillance" approach that uses natural supplements to either prevent cancer from ever developing, or prevent existing prostate cancer from growing and spreading outside the prostate. https://www.youtube.com/watch?v=oms4ZdDcvJl

In this video, Dr. Katz talks about how inflammation can lead to cancer. Therefore, one can reduce their risk of cancer by reducing inflammation. Medication that is designed to block inflammation can have severe side effects. Therefore, it is better to try a natural diet. It is known that a high fat diet can lead to inflammation in the body, so therefore, one should eat a low fat diet. Dr. Katz studied Zyflamend, a natural supplement consisting of 10 herbs, including ginger, turmeric, green tea, and holy basil. The herbs in Zyflamend can interfere with the inflammation pathway, and therefore reduce inflammation. Indeed, it has been used successfully to treat arthritis. But it can also lower PSA. A phase 1 clinical trial at Columbia University demonstrated that Zyflamend can reduce inflammation, and perhaps therefore help prevent the precancerous condition PIN from developing into prostate cancer. The study also found Zyflamend had no side effects, if it is taken with food. https://www.youtube.com/watch?v=xbj42gQNKml

In this video, we see that gluten can cause inflammation. Also sugars, even natural ones in fruit, can also cause inflammation of the liver and water retention. Apparently, there is a simple test to see if there is inflammation in your body: simply squeeze your wrist - you should feel bone. If you feel a layer of fluid, this indicates water retention, and hence inflammation in the body.

http://www.mayoclinic.org/healthy-lifestyle/nutrition-and-healthy-eating/in-depth/gluten-free-diet/art-20048530

Here you can read about a gluten-free diet. Gluten is a protein that is found in grains such as wheat, barley, rye. Many healthy food are gluten free, such as beans, seeds, nuts, eggs, fish, fruits, vegetables, corn, buckwheat, quinoa, rice, and soy.

Case Study 9 —

The conventional treatment of Androgen Deprivation Therapy (ADT) has many documented successes in treating prostate cancer, but also some downsides as well.

There was a small group study of seventy-three men, average age of sixty-seven, with average PSA of 9, including both medium and high risk cases. After twelve years, 29 percent never required further treatment, while 33 percent required periodic ADT to keep PSA less than 5. Other patients chose to undergo surgery or radiation therapy. Only three men died within three, eight, and eleven years after taking ADT [Cohen, p. 106-107]. Therefore, forty-five men of the sixty-seven (62 percent) never needed any surgery, radiation, or any other invasive treatment. This gave me great motivation to begin hormone therapy.

Because ADT works by depriving the body of testosterone, one can experience downsides such as less of muscle mass, hot flashes, pain, extremely vivid dreams (in my case)... Of course, the side effects vary with each person. Here are three ADT success stories:

1) A man with a PSA of 34 and a Gleason score of 6 had his PSA reduced to 0.3 while on ADT for only two months, and ADT was then discontinued. His cancer disappeared after two years.

2) In 1997, a seventy-eight year old man presented with a PSA of 33 and many palpable nodules in the prostate during the DRE, highly suggestive of prostate cancer, which a biopsy then confirmed. He went on ADT for a year and a half. In 2008, his PSA was still .6, and he was cancer free at the age of ninety.

3) In 1997, a sixty-four year old man presented with a PSA of 12. A biopsy found an area of intermediate grade cancer and two areas of low grade cancer in the prostate. After ADT for five months, his PSA was not detectable. Unfortunately, six years later, a biopsy showed that the cancer had returned. His PSA dropped after starting on ADT again. A repeat biopsy one year later showed that he was cancer free. Then ADT was stopped, and was stable as of 2009.

Case Study 10 —

Dr. Mirko Beljanski is a great scientist with great accomplishments. He developed a great theory about cancer and how to cure it. See [Walker] for a very well written book on his accomplishments. In the case studies below, we document many successful cancer cases cured using his products. Nowadays many notorious urologists, oncologists, and universities around the world flock to continue Dr. Beljanski's unfinished research projects.

In particular, in 2012, 177,489 were diagnosed with prostate cancer, and 27,244 died of prostate cancer – about 15 percent. It appears that the data is just a general picture, and we do not know the number of patients which were treated with conventional treatment, integrated therapy, or holistic treatment using only herbal supplements. Perhaps many top notch urologists or medical professors are afraid to be prosecuted by mainstream medicine companies, which may have a monopoly on medical treatment. According to Dr. Morton Walker, Dr. Beljanski's products have saved up to 5,000 patients as of 2013 [Walker, p.15]. The question is from 2004 to 2016, how many more patients of cancer and HIV have been saved by only Dr. Beljanski's products? Based on new technology and 3,500 members of CIRIS (Center of Innovation, Research and Scientific Information, an organization formed by users of Dr. Beljanski's supplements), the main question is, it is a linear or an exponential increase?

From there, one may ask: how many patients have been saved by all holistic or alternative therapies combined? At this moment, there are no statistics showing how many people have been saved by holistic or alternative therapy in 2012, so while many urologists may claim that only a small amount have been saved by traditional therapy, the reality is that we cannot know. Please, read the following websites.

http://www.naturalnews.com/027020_cancer_AMA_treatment.html
http://www.lifeextension.com/magazine/2012/7/wellness-profile/page-01
http://www.naturopathic.org/content.asp?contentid=505
http://drsircus.com/medicine/cancer/amazing-cancer-therapy-wipes-prostate-bone-cancer
http://www.burtongoldberg.com/alternativeprostatecancertreatmentoptions.html

Today, many students at graduate and medical schools are interested in researching cancer for their master's theses and doctorate dissertations.

Students are the catalyst for many universities to offer master and Ph.D. programs in cancer research. See, for example:

http://pathology.columbia.edu/education/graduate/

https://molgen.osu.edu/research-scholarship-opportunities

https://www.mdanderson.org/education-and-research/education-and-training/schools-and-programs/graduate-school-of-biomedical-sciences/index.html

http://drexel.edu/medicine/Academics/Graduate-School/Cancer-Biology/

http://www.wakehealth.edu/Research/Cancer-Biology/Graduate-Program.htm

http://www.cancerbiology.usf.edu/

http://www.umassmed.edu/gsbs/prospective-students/cancer-biology/program-overview/

http://www.ucdenver.edu/academics/colleges/medicalschool/departments/Pathology/academicprograms/cancerbiology/Pages/cancerbiologyprogram.aspx

https://medicine.umich.edu/medschool/education/phd-programs/about-pibs/programs/cancer-biology

http://www.utu.fi/en/news/news/Pages/award-winning-mathematical-model-predicts-adverse-events-of-chemotherapy-in-metastatic-prostate-cancer.aspx

The more outstanding cancer researchers there are, the more chances there are for traditional MDs to discover more knowledge and open their minds to the many directions there are for treating cancer, and therefore increase a cancer patient's chance for survival. I, the author, only try to do research online, and I do not have any professional opinion about the accuracy of information that I found on Google. Therefore, I do not have any legal responsibility.

As for Dr. Beljanski, I do not have many reservations or doubts that he is a scholar and that his products are helpful. Indeed, Dr. Beljanski took and showed extreme care about minute details – he was very precise and thorough. Ironically, he knew more than his boss on the subject of DNA and RNA, but he did not get the Nobel Prize, even though his research was a revolutionary discovery at his time. The sad thing is that people who knew less than him got the Nobel Prize during his time. Moreover, he understood well how DNA responded when exposed to carcinogens from the surrounding environment, as well as how to deal with that situation.

I attest that I am not an extremist with respect to any aspect of medicine. I always believe that every doctor, pharmaceutical company, and medical organization has a common interest: save as many human lives as possible.

Case Study 11 —

See *Cancer's Cause, Cancer's Cure* by Hugo House Publishers, 2011, p. 147–149 (Reprinted with permission). In April of 2004, a tiny bump that looked just like a pimple appeared on the thigh of Madame Elaine Escalon, in France. Unfortunately, a skin biopsy diagnosed melanoma. While chemotherapy is used to treat melanoma that has spread, as it had in her case, not everyone can be cured. Some patients have a life expectancy of less than nine months. Madame Escalon's story is as follows:

During a hospital stay, Madame Escalon encountered a woman who had been given the same death sentence by an oncologist, and yet conquered her own cancer, living in full health to date through the use of Dr. Beljanski's herbal products. Intrigued by this, Madame Escalon got more details on how to get the products.

After this, she was operated on to remove some of the melanoma. The surgeon cut out a nearly one-inch long tumor, along with surrounding tissue, thus leaving a hole in her thigh with the circumference of a grapefruit. Just two days later, she ordered Ginkgo Biloba supplements at the advice of her homeopathic doctor. She took 9 pills a day for two months and four pills a day of other Beljanski products for ten months.

After two months of suffering, her wound from surgery healed so quickly, with no need for a skin graft - this astonished her doctor. Her husband also took Gingko Biloba when he had bladder surgery. No surprise, his incision also healed quickly. Even to this date, her melanoma is in remission, which she believes is due to Dr. Beljanski's products, as she described in her taped testimonials. Today, Mrs. Escalon still takes Dr. Beljanski's products every spring and fall. She is a member of the CIRIS organization (a French organization of about 3000 people using Dr. Beljanski's products).

Case Study 12 —

See *Cancer's Cause, Cancer's Cure* by Hugo House Publishers, 2011 (Reprinted with permission.) Mr. Yvon Papineau had been a professional French fisherman since he was just fourteen years old. He sold his boat to go into semi-retirement as a regional supervisor of several fisheries.

He was keeping his health in good shape well into his seventies by biking every day or doing some other form of daily exercise. Then one day while biking, he experienced a pain in his throat, and his wife noticed a white oval object about the size of a pigeon egg inside the back of his throat.

The next day he saw his family doctor and got a prescription for antibiotics, which did not help. His doctor then sent him to an ear-nose-throat doctor, who tried yet another antibiotic. Nothing worked, and the pain intensified. He returned to the ENT doctor. Now concerned, the doctor operated on his throat, and unfortunately discovered a serious stage III malignancy which had metastasized to his mouth, throat, tonsil, and neck... It was very sad news for Mr. Papineau because his prognosis was to survive no more than twenty weeks, according to medical records. It was unfair to Mr. Papineau because he never was a smoker!

The clinician gave him twenty radiation treatments for twenty days, and then six chemotherapy sessions. The doctor's sad assessment was that he could die within three to six months. Actually, Mr. Papineau took Dr. Beljanski's products throughout his conventional treatment. The supplements protected him from the negative side effects of the radiation and chemotherapy. Furthermore, all the metastasized cancer cells were destroyed. Finally, his throat cancer disappeared at the end of one year. "Those Beljanski pills are part of my regular daily food supply, and they will remain so as long as I live," said Mr. Papineau.

Case Study 13 —

See *Cancer's Cause, Cancer's Cure* by Hugo House Publishers, 2011 (Reprinted with permission). This is the story of Monsieur Gerard Weidlich, a retired law enforcement officer – Chief Inspector with *Compagnie Republicaine de securite* (CRS). His main duty was to rescue near drowning victims.

In August 1985, he was infected with HIV-1. According to medical records at the time, his life expectancy was from two to five years. He took conventional medicine for AIDS patients at that time, but it did not work. Moreover, within a few months, he experienced many symptoms of AIDS such as herpes, and yeast infections from the fungus *Candida albicans*. AZT (azidothymidine) was the newest drug to be offered to him, but he refused.

He was lucky to get assistance from a group of AIDS patients, and from then on, he took Beljanski products, and thanks to those products, they saved his life from 1986 to 2007. Unfortunately, in 2007, he died due to a blockage in one of the main arteries in the lung, the same reason his mother died.

Case Study 14 —

I give thanks to the many cancer patients and medical scholars who have shared their experiences, frustrations, and triumphs when dealing with cancer. Perhaps your voices are the catalysts to drive medical research forward. Yes, the search for a prostate cancer cure, while minimizing side effects, encourages participation from many sources: prostate cancer scholars, traditional pharmaceutical companies, government funds, charitable organizations, medical schools,...

This is the case of Ai Hoa, a seventy-eight year old lady from Indonesia. In May of 2008, she had chocolate colored vaginal discharge. After many consultations with gynecologists, she was diagnosed with micro invasive squamous cell cancer (skin cancer) inside of her cervix. On March 25, 2009, she had twenty-eight dosages of radiation therapy and 3 dosages of brachytherapy.

The results were not useful, with many side-effects, and she returned to Penang on April 4, 2010. She decided to give up conventional treatments, and thought about another method of treatment. She took herbal treatments and juice therapy to about May 5, 2012. Her health was restored after this natural treatment.

Case Study 15 —

See *Cancer's Cause, Cancer's Cure* by Hugo House Publishers, 2011 (Reprinted with permission). Professor Boiteux, Ph.D., retired Professor of Physics at the University of Paris, is the only patient in the world, as far as I know, to have never adopted any conventional treatment, and instead only depended on Beljanski's medicine to put his prostate cancer into remission. Of course, he conquered the battlefield of his prostate cancer [Walker, pp. 111-119].

Professor Boiteux was also a former Director of Research at the CNRS (Centre National de la Recherche Scientifique or National Center for Scientific Research, France, http://www.cnrs.fr/en/home/faq.htm), which is the French equivalent to the National Institute of Health in the USA. He studied various treatments of most types of diseases, and in particular cancer.

In 1994, his local urologist gave him the bad news that he had prostate cancer at the age of seventy-three. The cancer was inoperable. Professor Boiteux listened to a colleague's advice to find a therapist who practiced CAIM (Complementary Alternative and Integrative Medicine).

Professor Boiteux only used two of Beljanski's products. One was powdered golden leaf ginkgo extract (Ginkgo V), and the other was an unnamed prescription, which I surmise is branded as Prostabel today. Even with his great knowledge of medicine, he nevertheless chose only the natural products developed by Dr. Mirko Beljanski to cure his prostate cancer. Moreover, the product also cured his osteoarthritis. He knew the many flaws in the conventional treatments for prostate cancer. Even many world famous medical institutes may make mistakes when deciding the best course of action for treatment.

7

Inflammation And Oxidative Stress

One potential cause of prostate cancer is ignoring oxidative and inflammatory stress. Oxidative stress is basically an imbalance in the body between the production of free radicals and the ability of the body to detoxify itself of these free radicals. Inflammation is a localized protective response to injury or irritants, the purpose of which is to destroy the injured tissue or irritant. Inflammatory stress and oxidative stress go hand in hand to cause various diseases in our bodies. Urologists consider them as predecessors of prostatic intraepithelial neoplasia (PIN), which is essentially a precancerous overgrowth of epithelial cells in the prostate. PIN is not detectable in a digital rectal examination, and does not raise PSA levels. Therefore, the condition is usually only discovered in a biopsy.

How then should we neutralize PIN, or prevent it altogether? Naturopathic physicians may have some clue to answer this question, as they are rigorously trained just like urologists are, see for example, http://aanmc.org/resources/curriculum.

There are several risk factors for prostate cancer.

1) Age is one, prostate cancer is rare in men under 40, but the risk for prostate cancer increases steeply after age 50.

2) Race: prostate cancer occurs in more in African-American men, and less in Asian and Hispanic men.

3) Family history: having a father or brother with the disease more than doubles your risk.

4) Sexually transmitted diseases can lead to inflammation of the prostate, and therefore increase the risk of prostate cancer.

5) Some studies have shown that obese men may be at higher risk for advanced or aggressive prostate cancer.

6) There have been some studies into the connection between diet and prostate cancer. A diet high in red meat with high-fat dairy products and less fruits and vegetables can raise your risk for prostate cancer.

7) Being exposed to certain chemicals, such as Agent Orange, can also increase your risk for prostate cancer.
   (Sources: http://www.cancer.org/cancer/prostatecancer/detailedguide/prostate-cancer-risk-factors and http://www.publichealth.va.gov/exposures/agentorange/conditions/prostate_cancer.asp)

Perhaps by preventing the precancerous condition PIN, we can thus prevent prostate cancer. Moreover, Dr. Mirko Beljanski studied how carcinogens work at the DNA level to cause cancer to develop in the body. See [Walker] for more information.

8

When Is A Prostate Biopsy Really Necessary?

As you have seen, my prostate biopsy was not the most pleasant experience. So then, how do we decide when a prostate biopsy is really necessary? That is, at what age does a "watch and wait" approach result in a similar outcome to choosing the biopsy route? This is especially relevant to me, as I was age seventy-five at the time.

Urologists and oncologists use factors such as the patient's health history and current health, results of the DRE exam, age, PSA, ... to determine if a prostate biopsy is necessary. The ultimate goal of a prostate biopsy is to determine the Gleason score of the prostate cancer. From there, the patient's risk is calculated to be low, intermediate, or high. See, for example, http://www.cancer.org/cancer/prostatecancer/detailedguide/prostate-cancer-staging

After the determination of Gleason score and risk level, the urologist and oncologist can now suggest treatment options.

Thanks to the technological advances that medical researchers make, nowadays we have many more tests to use before rushing to perform the rather invasive procedure of prostate biopsy, which can have some side effects. For example, I had blood in both my urine and stool for days after my biopsy.

There are many advanced medical imaging techniques (non-invasive) such as the Dynamic Contrast Enhanced (DCE) MRI, the Color Doppler

Ultrasound, and the Carbon-11 Acetate PET/CT scan that can give clearer pictures of the prostate and surrounding tissue. The Color Doppler Ultrasound can also lead to a more accurate staging and prognosis, although it has limitations of detecting prostate cancer which is smaller than 5 millimeters.

In addition, there are several tests which are based on genomics/DNA/RNA, and other cellular level characteristics such as ConfirmMDX, Polaris, OncotypeDX, ProstaVysion, Decipher Test, and the Caris Molecular Intelligence Profile and Profile Plus. However, these tests need a sample of prostate tissue. Nevertheless, they can help give a more accurate level of risk to avoid over-treatment of men with less aggressive cancers. See [Katz] for more information on these tests. You can also see http://advancedcancerresearchinstitute.com/advanced-cancer-diagnostics-detection-and-monitoring-free-info/ for more advanced, non-invasive tests. I had a dilemma whether or not to take those tests. The first reason is the reliability of these tests is not clear, as they are just too new. Secondly, there is no concrete scientific evidence for these tests so far.

Unfortunately, even when urologists and oncologists combine all tests so far, the degree of reliability is probably around 90 percent. Moreover, medical imaging may have difficulty to determine whether cancerous lesions are inside or outside the prostate. Therefore, I wonder if it possible to use Morse Theory (a generalization of multivariable calculus) to accurately parameterize a three dimensional object by assembling two dimensional cross-sections. However, these imaging tests are not yet accepted to replace prostate biopsies. In addition, I would have to be exposed to radiation when taking these tests. Comparing the benefits and risks, I decided to take the prostate biopsy if all my famous urologists and oncologists could not come up with another approach for their second opinion.

Secondly, I wonder why not use the amount of PIN in prostate biopsy tissue. Perhaps knowing the amount of PIN can help determine treatment options. As PIN is considered a precancerous growth, PIN may be one factor to decide if the wait and see approach is appropriate.

9

A Few Thoughts

Chapter 6 motivated me to search and experiment for a solution to my prostate cancer with Gleason score 8. First, I found some hope for an alternate approach to put my prostate cancer in remission in Dr. Katz's book [Katz]: *Dr. Katz's Guide to Prostate Health From Conventional to Holistic Therapies* (ISBN: 978-1893910379).

The next book [Cohen] I found was *Prostate Cancer Breakthroughs 2014: New Tests, New Treatments, Better Options: A Step-by-Step Guide to Cutting-Edge Diagnostic Tests and 12 Medically-Problem Treatments* by Dr. Jay S. Cohen (ISBN: 978-0988710504), and this book motivated me to begin hormone therapy with Lupron. Lupron is a form of androgen deprivation therapy, which is based on the fact that prostate cancer cells need male hormones (androgens), like testosterone, to grow. The medical community believes that androgen deprivation therapy slows the speed of prostate cancer cell growth and may also shrink the tumor. In Dr. Cohen's book, I learned that many patients with both intermediate and high risk prostate cancer never needed any further treatment after their initial course of ADT, and this was great encouragement for me.

The next three books allowed me to formulate my own alternate treatment for my prostate cancer. One was *Cancer's Cause, Cancer's Cure: The Truth about Cancer, It's Causes, Cures, and Prevention* by Morton Walker, DPM (ISBN: 978-1936449101). The next two [Goldstone1, Goldstone2] were both by Daniel J. Goldstone, who was able to put his prostate cancer in full

47

remission with his holistic approach: *I Beat Cancer Holistically: Protocols for Breast, Colon, Lung, and Prostate Cancer* (ISBN: 978-1600477836), *Advanced Prostate Cancer and Me: How I Reduced my PSA 100% Holistically* (ISBN: 978-1441502247). Mr. Goldstone's story gave me very strong motivation to take a holistic approach, in addition to hormone therapy.

As a reader and a learner, I thank Dr. Morton Walker, DPM who devoted his time to write Chapter 8 of his book [Morton]. I have no opinion on the Beljanski remedy dosages as suggested by the French physician, Christian Marcowith, MD. However, I do have an opinion on Chapter 7 of "Cancer Prevention". In fact, I prefer Chapter 7 of "Diet Whole Foods and Supplement," p. 165 - 219 of [Katz]. His strategy is to choose organic over non-organic foods and eliminate red meat consumption. He advocates eating wild caught salmon and shrimp. I guess, Dr. Katz's conventional wisdom is rather safe when compared to other supplements. Nevertheless, each individual must know which foods and supplements are suitable for their own bodies. Therefore, in general, one is entirely responsible for his or her own choices of diet and supplements.

I also try to keep up with new developments and research in prostate cancer, by any means possible, such as searching the Internet, and consulting with authorities in prostate cancer. Using the Internet, I investigated and researched what supplements could reduce oxidative stress and inflammatory stress. Readers should know that information on the Internet is not a reliable source of medical information. Readers should do their own research and take responsibility for evaluating the information that they find before they select their own holistic supplements for treating prostate cancer.

Nếu độc giả biết đọc tiếng Việt hay là người Việt Nam, xin mời độc giả đọc 16 bài chiến thuật và chiến lược; môn học sở trường của tôi. Nhờ thế, tôi đã áp dụng môn sở trường nầy để tự đi tìm giải pháp đánh bại bệnh terminal prostate cancer.

If you can read Vietnamese, you can also read sixteen articles that I have written with the purpose of teaching tactics and strategy. Knowledge of tactics and strategy allowed me to create a plan to beat my prostate cancer.

- Chiến Thuật và Chiến Lược

  http://www.generalhieu.com/thuong_chienthuat_chienluoc.htm

- Chiến Thuật và Chiến Lược - Phần 2
  http://www.generalhieu.com/thuong_chienthuat_chienluoc_2.htm
- Chiến Thuật và Chiến Lược - Phần 3
  http://www.generalhieu.com/thuong_chienthuat_chienluoc_3.htm
- Tổ Chức, Lãnh Đạo và Chiến Lược- Chiến Thuật Hành Động
  http://www.generalhieu.com/thuong_chienthuat_chienluoc_4.htm
- Chiến Thuật và Chiến Lược - Phần 5
  http://www.generalhieu.com/thuong_chienthuat_chienluoc_5.htm
- Chiến Thuật và Chiến Lược - Phần 6
  http://www.generalhieu.com/thuong_chienthuat_chienluoc_6.htm
- Chiến Thuật và Chiến Lược - Phần 7
  http://www.generalhieu.com/thuong_chienthuat_chienluoc_7.htm
- Chiến Thuật và Chiến Lược - Phần 8
  http://www.generalhieu.com/thuong_chienthuat_chienluoc_8.htm
- Chiến Thuật và Chiến Lược - Phần 9
  http://www.generalhieu.com/thuong_chienthuat_chienluoc_9.htm
- Chiến Thuật và Chiến Lược - Phần 10
  http://www.generalhieu.com/thuong_chienthuat_chienluoc_10.htm
- Chiến Thuật và Chiến Lược - Phần 11
  http://www.generalhieu.com/thuong_chienthuat_chienluoc_11.htm
- Chiến Thuật và Chiến Lược - Phần 12
  http://www.generalhieu.com/thuong_chienthuat_chienluoc_12.htm
- Chiến Thuật và Chiến Lược - Phần 13
  http://www.generalhieu.com/thuong_chienthuat_chienluoc_13.htm
- Chiến Thuật và Chiến Lược - Phần 14
  http://www.generalhieu.com/thuong_chienthuat_chienluoc_14.htm
- Chiến Thuật và Chiến Lược - Phần 15
  http://www.generalhieu.com/thuong_chienthuat_chienluoc_15.htm
- Chiến Thuật và Chiến Lược - Phần 16
  http://www.generalhieu.com/thuong_chienthuat_chienluoc_16.htm

- Chiến Thuật và Chiến Lược - Phần 17
  http://www.generalhieu.com/thuong_chienthuat_chienluoc_17.htm
- Chiến Thuật và Chiến Lược - Phần 18
  http://www.generalhieu.com/thuong_chienthuat_chienluoc_18.htm

Example:

Năm 1975 CSVN thắng lợi chiến thuật và chiến lược hạn chế vì chiếm đoạt toàn thể lãnh thổ VNCH, nhưng chưa thắng được chiến lược toàn diện về phương diện chiến lược. Tại sao? Phải có hai điều kiện để chiến thắng chiến lược toàn diện. Đó là làm chủ diện địa và tiêu diệt ý chí chiến đấu địch.

Trong thực tế, Quân-Cán-Dân vẫn còn giữ vững lá cờ vàng, tổ chức các cuộc biểu tình chống CSVN, chống đối NQ 36 CSVN, phản đối kế hoạch kết nghĩa thành phố Irwin-Nha Trang, ...Vì vậy hiện tượng Irwin chứng tỏ CSVN chưa tiêu diệt được ý chí của chúng ta.

Explanation: The communists have occupied the territory of the Republic of Vietnam from 1975 until today. In fact, while they have conquered the Republic of Vietnam in a tactical sense, they have not conquered it in a strategic sense. This is because they still cannot destroy the political will and communication of the South Vietnamese people. This analogy can also be extended to one's battle against prostate cancer. For example, a prostate cancer patient may win tactically against prostate cancer by choosing the invasive treatment option of surgery, or radiation therapy to lower PSA. Of course, he has won tactically when PSA drops below 1 point. However, the problem is that PSA may have a chance to rise up again. In this case, the patient has lost strategically. Winning strategically means that the PSA must never climb again. Case studies 11-15 in Chapter 6 are examples of using an integrated strategy to achieve a strategic victory against cancer. Moreover, changing your diet to reduce inflammation and carcinogens can also help to achieve a strategic victory.

10

Impact Of My Integrative Approach—From Diagnosis To Remission

The goal of my selection of herbs and supplements is to reduce my PSA. Moreover, I thank Dr. Beljanski, Dr. Aaron Katz, Dr. Morton Walker, and Mr. Daniel Goldstone for their books and research. I learned from their lists of herbs and non-traditional supplements which paved the way for me to develop my own lists for my personal use. In addition to the supplements mentioned in Chapter 5, thanks to Dr. Katz's book [Katz], I am taking some more supplements from New Chapter (Zyflamend Prostate, Every Man's One Daily 40+ Multivitamin, and Prostate 5LX).

Please, remember that some people may feel that some of my choices are not helpful for their particular situation. In this case, one should eliminate the offending supplement right away, and choose another supplement that is compatible with their body, in consultation with a natural doctor.

There are several reasons why I chose to take Lupron hormone therapy.

1. The MRI showed that I had metastatic cancer, and it had spread to my pelvic bone.
2. The result of my PSA test.
3. I am over seventy-five years old.
4. I was exposed to Agent Orange in the jungle for over ten years.

5. I was exposed to too much radiation prior to 1975 because of military missions, and exposed to too much radiation in the form of X-rays after 1975.

6. My Gleason score was greater than 8, which is classified as "high risk".

I initially planned to take aggressive treatment such as surgery or radiation, but decided against this thanks to the advice of all my competent urologists from OU Cancer Center, Mayo Clinic in Arizona, and UT Southwestern Medical Center in Dallas. I spent a lot of time to come up with my best option, and I finally settled on an integrated approach. I decided to combine Lupron hormone therapy together with herbs and supplements. I believed that I was on the right path. For many months prior to beginning hormone therapy in January of 2016, I was suffering pain in my pelvic bone (worse on the left side) and having difficulty sleeping at night. I decided to buy some herbs and supplements for an experimental trial, starting on February 10, 2016, and ending on May 20, 2016. After starting the supplements, I began to sleep well again. Moreover, after one month, the pain in my pelvic bone had disappeared. I know that many people can experience rather heavy side effects of hormone therapy, but I was fortunate to only experience one: I had some vivid dreams and delusions at night for a brief period of time. However, these disappeared as my health improved. I began to regain my balance, and I no longer experienced any pain when walking in the morning, a part of my daily exercise routine.

At this time, I feel my health is now better than it was in 2009 when I retired. Therefore, I do not regret my integrative approach. Of course, I could be deceiving myself with feelings of good health, but PSA tests don't lie! I was on Lupron for three months: from January 22, 2016 to April 22, 2016. Below is a table showing the change in my PSA over time.

Date	Total PSA (ng/mL)	Free PSA (ng/mL)
10/02/2015	15.90	1.57
03/30/2016	2.7	Not tested
04/21/2016	1.5	Not tested
05/16/2016	0.95	0.20

On March 30, 2016, I took a PSA test and found my total PSA had dropped from 15.9 to 2.7 (an 83% reduction). Then a PSA test on April 21, 2016 showed that my total PSA had fallen from 2.7 to 1.5 (a 45% reduction). On 05/16/2016, a PSA test showed a total PSA of 0.95 (a 37% reduction) and a free PSA of 0.20. This proved to me that my alternate therapy was contributing significantly to reduce my PSA, because Lupron alone does not produce such a steep drop in PSA. See the end of the chapter for documentation.

Here are two informative links about PSA testing:

https://zerocancer.org/learn/psa-testing

http://www.harvardprostateknowledge.org/what-is-the-difference-between-psa-and-free-psa

As a protein produced by the prostate, PSA in the bloodstream can either be bound to other proteins or on its own (unbounded). Free PSA is a measurement of the unbounded PSA. Total PSA simply measures the amount of bound and unbound PSA together. Apparently, the ratio of free PSA to total PSA is correlated with the probability that a man has prostate cancer. A higher ratio corresponds to a lower risk of prostate cancer. So, the greater percentage of free PSA, the better. In the literature, the correlation is only claimed for men with total PSA between 4.0 to ng/mL to 10 ng/mL. Nevertheless, perhaps this correlation extends to men with total PSA outside of the 4.0 to 10.0 ng/mL interval. For completeness, we present the table below.

% of free PSA (when total PSA is between 4.0-10.0 ng/mL)	Probability of prostate cancer
0% – 10%	56%
10% – 15%	28%
15% – 20%	20%
20% – 25%	16%
Greater than 25%	8%

Source: Journal of the American Medical Association, May 20, 1998.

As you can see from my PSA testing, in October of 2015, my free PSA percentage was 1.57/15.9 = 9.9%. But in May of 2016, the free PSA percentage had risen to 0.2/0.95 = 21.1%. Thus my free PSA percentage has more than doubled. It is not clear or certain if the above table can be used to infer probabilities, because the total PSA in each case is outside of the 4.0-10.0 ng/mL interval. Nevertheless, the fact that the free PSA percentage has more than doubled is a very good sign. More concretely, the total amount of PSA is below 1.0 ng/mL. A safe range for PSA is between 0 to 2.5 ng/mL. This, taken together with my good feelings of health (eating, exercising, and sleeping well), allows me to conclude that my prostate cancer is in remission.

At this moment, I need to test the impacts of Lupron hormone therapy, herbs, and supplements. So, I may stop testing my PSA for a while, and listen to my body every day. If my pain ever comes back, then I will have to do blood tests again. If my pain continues to stay away, I will definitely continue to take my selection of herbs and supplements. Someday I will have to test my PSA again, and perhaps some other test to monitor the status of my body, and prove that I have won on the battlefield against prostate cancer. One advantage of my protocol for treating prostate cancer is that I do not need prescriptions for drugs at a pharmacy. My strategy is self-observation for any changes in my body when I begin taking the supplements, so that I may either increase dosage, reduce dosage, or eliminate the supplement altogether.

By no means do I think conventional therapy is useless, as it is the end result of years of scientific research. But if you decide to pursue conventional therapy, why exclude alternative treatments? Indeed, perhaps a combination of the two would provide the best outcome. Intuitively this would be the case, and a 1971 paper of Beljanski confirmed this to be the case (also see [Walker, p.125]). The paper describes experiments on lymphoma in mice. The experiment considered four groups of mice, those with no treatment, only chemotherapy, only Beljanksi's *Raowolfia vomitoria* extract, and finally a combination of chemotherapy and *Raowolfia* extract. Those receiving no treatment all died within a month, as one would expect. Of those who received chemotherapy alone, 45% were alive at 90 days and of those who received *Raowolfia* alone, 30% were alive at 90 days. Unexpectedly, those who received both treatments *all survived.*

At this time (4/12/16), my PSA has almost been reduced to zero, but I do not believe that PSA is the only factor to decide that my prostate cancer of Gleason score 8 has been cured. There are many factors that contribute to the answer to the question: "How to decide when prostate cancer has been cured completely?" Maybe hormone therapy is the answer? Maybe it is the supplements that I took? Maybe it is my exercise daily? Maybe I should listen to my body every day? Maybe there are other factors? Most likely it is a combination of many factors. Perhaps I should consult my oncologist and urologist on the strategy of "waiting and watching"? Perhaps I may also try one of the advanced tests for cancer mentioned in Chapter 8.

But I do know this. My positive attitude and absolute belief that I could handle my prostate cancer is what carried me through and has kept me alive.

```
Printed: 10/07/15  -0848       N o r m a n   R e g i o n a l              Page: 1
Norman Regional Hospital       Laboratory Services         James W. Seay, MD, FCAP
Moore Medical Center                                    Stephen C. Ingels, MD, FCAP
Healthplex Laboratory                                     Eric J. Thompson, MD, FCAP
Robinson Medical Plaza                                  Robert S. Littlejohn, MD, FCAP

Patient: THUONG,TRAN V                      Location: NLAB      Room:
Age/Sex: 75/MALE          Acct#:            Ord Phys: Ray,Michael T, DO
    DOB:                  MR#:              Copies To: Ray,Michael T, DO

Specimen #: 1002:RS00001R          Collected: 10/02/15 0719         Status: COMPLETE
Ordered:    PSA FR AND TTL

   [ H = High   L = Low   ** = Abnormal  * = Critical   # = Significant Change ]

        Test         |      Normal      |     Abnormal     |Flg|    Reference    |Loc


   PSA FR AND TTL    |                  |                  |   |                 |
     TOTAL PSA       |                  |       15.90      | H |0.00-2.50 NG/ML  |RML
     FREE PSA        |                  |        1.57      | H |0.00-0.41 NG/ML  |RML
                     |  Test performed at RML Tulsa
                     |  4142 S Mingo Rd, Tulsa OK 74146
                     |  CLIA# 37D2031514, Cindi Starkey, MD - Lab Director

RML - REGIONAL MEDICAL LABORATORY
     Regional Medical Laboratory
     1923 S. Utica Ave, Tulsa, OK 74104-6502
```

LabCorp

Patient Report

Specimen ID: 090-298-3820-0   Acct #:   Phone: (954) 485-3322   Rte: 28
Control ID: 25908087

THUONG, TRAN VAN

Health Testing Centers
2760 W. OAKLAND PARK BLVD.
FORT LAUDERDALE FL 33311

(405) 310-4404

Patient Details	**Specimen Details**	**Physician Details**
DOB:	Date collected: 03/30/2016 1428 Local	Ordering: C DAVIS
Age(y/m/d): 075	Date entered: 03/30/2016	Referring:
Gender: M SSN:	Date reported: 04/01/2016 0818 Local	ID: 1144360256
Patient ID:		NPI: 1144360256

General Comments & Additional Information
Alternate Control Number: 25908087
Total Volume: Not Provided
Alternate Patient ID: Not Provided
Fasting: No

Ordered Items
PAP + PSA; Venipuncture

TESTS	RESULT	FLAG	UNITS	REFERENCE INTERVAL	LAB
PAP + PSA					
Prostatic Acid Phos, Serum	1.6		ng/mL	0.0 - 3.5	01
DPC Immulite 2000 methodology.					
Prostate Specific Ag, Serum	2.7		ng/mL	0.0 - 4.0	02

Roche ECLIA methodology.
According to the American Urological Association, Serum PSA should
decrease and remain at undetectable levels after radical
prostatectomy. The AUA defines biochemical recurrence as an initial
PSA value 0.2 ng/mL or greater followed by a subsequent confirmatory
PSA value 0.2 ng/mL or greater.
Values obtained with different assay methods or kits cannot be used
interchangeably. Results cannot be interpreted as absolute evidence
of the presence or absence of malignant disease.

01	BN	LabCorp Burlington	Dir: William F Hancock, MD
		1447 York Court, Burlington, NC 27215-3361	
02	DA	LabCorp Dallas	Dir: CN Etufugh, MD
		7777 Forest Lane Suite C350, Dallas, TX 75230-2544	

For Inquiries, the physician may contact Branch: **800-762-4344** Lab: **972-598-6000**

Date Issued: 04/01/16 0949 ET   **FINAL REPORT**   Page 1 of 1

LabCorp   **Patient Report**

Specimen ID: 112-298-1276-0   Acct #:   Phone: (954) 485-3322   Rte: 28
Control ID: 26375611

THUONG, TRAN VAN   Health Testing Centers
                                               2760 W. OAKLAND PARK BLVD.
                                               FORT LAUDERDALE FL 33311

(405) 310-4404

Patient Details	Specimen Details	Physician Details
DOB:	Date collected: 04/21/2016 0929 Local	Ordering: C DAVIS
Age(y/m/d): 076	Date entered: 04/21/2016	Referring:
Gender: M SSN:	Date reported: 04/23/2016 0911 Local	ID: 1144360256
Patient ID:		NPI: 1144360256

General Comments & Additional Information
Alternate Control Number: 26375611   Alternate Patient ID: Not Provided
Total Volume: Not Provided   Fasting: No

Ordered Items
PAP + PSA; Venipuncture

TESTS	RESULT	FLAG	UNITS	REFERENCE INTERVAL	LAB
PAP + PSA					
Prostatic Acid Phos, Serum	2.4		ng/mL	0.0 - 3.5	01
DPC Immulite 2000 methodology.					
Prostate Specific Ag, Serum	1.5		ng/mL	0.0 - 4.0	02

Roche ECLIA methodology.
According to the American Urological Association, Serum PSA should
decrease and remain at undetectable levels after radical
prostatectomy. The AUA defines biochemical recurrence as an initial
PSA value 0.2 ng/mL or greater followed by a subsequent confirmatory
PSA value 0.2 ng/mL or greater.
Values obtained with different assay methods or kits cannot be used
interchangeably. Results cannot be interpreted as absolute evidence
of the presence or absence of malignant disease.

01	BN	LabCorp Burlington	Dir: William F Hancock, MD
		1447 York Court, Burlington, NC 27215-3361	
02	DA	LabCorp Dallas	Dir: CN Etufugh, MD
		7777 Forest Lane Suite C350, Dallas, TX 75230-2544	

For inquiries, the physician may contact Branch: 800-762-4344 Lab: 972-598-6000

Date Issued: 04/23/16 0924 ET   **FINAL REPORT**   Page 1 of 1

[H = High   L = Low   ** = Abnormal   * = Critical   # = Significant Change]

Test	Normal	Abnormal	Flg	Reference	Loc
PSA FR AND TTL					
TOTAL PSA	0.95			0.00-2.50 ng/mL	RML
FREE PSA	0.20			0.00-0.41 ng/dL	RML

RML - REGIONAL MEDICAL LABORATORY
    Regional Medical Laboratory
    1923 S. Utica Ave, Tulsa, OK 74104-6502

References

[Cohen] Dr. Jay S. Cohen, *Prostate Cancer Breakthroughs 2014: New Tests, New Treatments, Better Options: A Step-by-Step Guide to Cutting-Edge Diagnostic Tests and 12 Medically-Problem Treatments*, ISBN: 978-0988710504 (also see Dr. Cohen's website: http://www. prostatecancerbreakthroughs.com)

[Goldstone1] Daniel J. Goldstone, *Advanced Prostate Cancer and Me: How I Reduced my PSA 100% Holistically*, ISBN: 978-1441502247

[Goldstone2] Daniel J. Goldstone, *I Beat Cancer Holistically: Protocols for Breast, Colon, Lung, and Prostate Cancer*, ISBN: 978-1600477836

[Guess] Guess, BW, et al., *Modified citrus pectin (MCP) increases the prostate-specific antigen doubling time in men with prostate cancer: a phase II pilot study.* Prostate Cancer Prostatic Dis, 2003;6(4): 301-4.

[Katz] Dr. Aaron E. Katz, *Dr. Katz's Guide to Prostate Health From Conventional to Holistic Therapies*, ISBN: 978-1893910379

[Reuter] Reuter, S., Gupta, Chaturvedi, and Aggarwal, *Oxidative stress, inflammation, and cancer: How are they linked?*, Free Radic Biol Med. 2010 Dec 1: 49(11): 1603-1616 (http://www.ncbi.nlm.nih.gov/pmc/articles/ PMC2990475/)

[Strum] Strum, S, et al. *Modified citrus pectin slows PSA doubling time: A pilot clinical trial.* International Conference on Diet and Prevention of Cancer. 1999. Tampere, Finland.

[Walker] Morton Walker, DPM, *Cancer's Cause, Cancer's Cure: The Truth about Cancer, It's Causes, Cures, and Prevention*, ISBN: 978-1936449101

Appendix

Here we compile useful resources and references. Many are academic, peer-reviewed articles which study anti-cancer properties of many of the supplements mentioned in the text. The articles are organized by subject matter.

Information about my military experience:
1. http://www.generalhieu.com/snoulthuong-2.htm
2. http://www.patriotfiles.com/archive/generalhieu/chinhnghia_arvn-2.htm

General information about Dr. Beljanski's discoveries:
3. "If you are undergoing chemotherapy or radiotherapy, you need to know about RNA-fragments"
4. "The Columbia Connection"
5. "How One Man's Courage is Helping Cancer Patients Across America"
6. "Golden Leaf Ginkgo Extract for Radiation Protection and Skin Fibrosis"
7. "Prostabel Reduces Men's PSA Counts" Source: *HealthyLivinG*
8. "Prostabel – Men's Serious Prostate Health Support" Source: *HealthyLivinG*

9. "High PSA, Negative Biopsy, Now What?"

10. "Extracts of Pao Pereira and Rauwolfia Vomitoria Show Promise to Enhance Prostate Health"
Source: http://www.townsendletter.com/July2012/walker0712.html

11. "Beljanski's Products" – A useful blogpost on Dr. Beljanski's products
Source: http://michelescancerblog.blogspot.com/2013/07/beljanski-products.html

AIDS and Dr. Beljanski's products:

12. "Cancer and AIDS the victory? The results of a thirty year research in molecular biology"
Source: http://www.whale.to/cancer/beljanski1.html

General information about choosing an approach to integrated treatment:

13. Source: http://www.self-helpcancer.org/

General information about holistic prostate treatments

14. "The Holistic Approach to Prostate Health"
Source: *Integrative Medicine, A Clinician's Journal*

Information about biomarker tests for detecting prostate cancer:

15. "New Biomarker Tests for Prostate Cancer"

Information about non invasive/non radiation tests for detecting cancer:

16. "Advanced Cancer Diagnostics, Early Detection and Reliable Monitoring"
Source: http://advancedcancerresearchinstitute.com/advanced-cancer-diagnostics-detection-and-monitoring-free-info/

Other people's battles with prostate cancer:

17. Charlie Redd
    Source: http://www.yananow.org/display_story.php?id=162

18. George Hardy
    Source: http://www.yananow.org/display_story.php?id=376

Academic (technical) articles on anti-cancer properties of *Pao Pereira/ Rauwolfia vomitoria:*

19. "Inhibition of pancreatic cancer and potentiation of gemcitabine effects by the extract of Pao Pereira"
    Source: *Oncology Reports*

20. "Pao Pereira Extract Suppresses Castration-Resistant Prostate Cancer Cell Growth, Survival, and Invasion Through Inhibition of NFkB Signaling"
    Source: *Integrative Cancer Therapies*

21. "Beta-Carboline Alkaloid-Enriched Extract from the Amazonian Rain Forest Tree Pao Pereira Suppresses Prostate Cancer Cells"
    Source: *Journal for the Society for Integrative Oncology*

22. "Two Herbal Extracts for Protecting Prostate Cell DNA"
    Source: *Integrative Medicine*

23. "Anti-prostate cancer activity of a beta-carboline alkaloid enriched extract from *Rauwolfia vomitoria*"
    Source: *International Journal of Oncology*

Important News for Chemotherapy and Radiotherapy Patients

Excerpted with permission from HealthyLivinG Magazine
(HealthyLivinGMagazine.us)

If you are undergoing chemotherapy or radiotherapy, you need to know about RNA-fragments.

A platelet is a colorless blood cell necessary for normal blood clotting; without them, the body has no secondary mechanism to stop internal bleeding. They also prevent the leakage of red blood cells from an uninjured blood vessel. By design, platelets are not long-lived in the body and usually are around only about nine days, so your body must constantly re-manufacture its platelets to replace those it loses.

This indifference to these colorless cells all change when people undergo chemotherapy or radiotherapy for cancer treatment. But why are platelet levels such a problem to cancer patients, anyway?

The normal blood platelet count ranges from 150,000 to 450,000 for every cubic millimeter of blood for a healthy individual. However, radiotherapy and chemotherapy attack not only cancer cells but also the body's healthy bone marrow, gastrointestinal tract, and mouth. The bone marrow is where blood cells are manufactured, and if the levels of platelets become too low, as they frequently do during chemotherapy or radiotherapy, treatment must be stopped.

Thrombocytopenia is when platelets are lost from the bloodstream faster than they can be replaced. "The result is that all of a sudden you get incredibly low levels of both white blood cells, for which we have some drugs now, and platelets, for which we can't do anything other than transfusions and wait," says Dr. James Grutsch, clinical trial consultant to the prestigious Cancer Treatment Centers of America (CTCA), a network of regional hospitals throughout the U.S. that is dedicated to fighting cancer with the very latest and most successful integrative tools from both conventional and complementary medicine.

Although the pharmaceutical industry has come up with drug that are able to help the body to maintain white blood cell counts, the same is not so for its platelets.

Many chemotherapy and radiotherapy protocols, which might otherwise have saved the lives of cancer patients, are halted at least temporarily because of dangerously low platelet counts, Dr. Grutsch told us. "It's a major problem in cancer treatment."

At the Cancer Treatment Centers of America, the oncologists and medical experts are constantly seeking out real ways to help patients fight back against cancer and get through their chemotherapy and radiotherapy.

RISING HOPE AND THE LANDMARK WORK OF MIRKO BELJANSKI, PhD

Ironically, in the late 1970s, Dr. Grutsch was a young researcher at the Pasteur Institute in Paris where the great molecular biologist Mirko Beljanski was one of the elite scientists peering into the very molecular secrets of life.

"In those days, the Pasteur Institute was the leading institute of molecular biology in the non-English-speaking world," Dr. Grutsch said. But Beljanski's research priorities came into direct conflict with those of Jacques Monad, the director of the institute, who claimed DNA to be an omnipotent molecule. Dr. Beljanski was pioneering research into ribonucleic acid (RNA) and proving RNA indeed spoke back to DNA and gave it new information that changed its blueprint. "Monad was brilliant, and like many brilliant people, if you did not follow his lead he could be very difficult to work with. The French researchers were in those days very driven and worked very hard and were very competitive." Dr. Grutsch told us. "I read his work, though, and I thought about it. Beljanski was right on target, and if he survived all those years under a director like Monad—who did not tolerate dummies—he must have been a darn good scientist. He had done all of the work to show us that we could actually save lives with RNA."

In 1969, Dr. Beljanski discovered small RNAs that transmitted hereditary characters absent in the DNA. In 1974, he became the first biologist to detect reverse transcriptase in bacteria. He then went on to find a technique to produce small primer-RNAs capable of helping bone marrow stem cells accelerate the production of white blood cells and platelets when many of these cells have been destroyed by conventional chemotherapy or radio-therapy. Currently, all the data show that these RNA fragments work only on the DNA of healthy cells, never that of cancer cells.

In 1979 in the peer-reviewed journal Experimental Cell Biology (47;3:218-25), Dr. Beljanski reported that ribosomal RNA from Escherichia coli is fragmented by pancreatic ribonuclease, leading to the appearance of particular RNA fragments. 'Some of these fragments act as primers for in vitro replication of DNA extracted from blood cell and platelet-forming tissues."

They restored "in a rapid and harmless way, normal circulating leukocyte and platelet levels when these have been drastically decreased by various chemotherapeutic agents mainly used in anticancer therapy. Imbalance between polynuclear and lymphocyte count…by cyclophosphamide can be rapidly corrected by treating…with active RNA fragments."

FINALLY, PLATELET SUPPORT FOR CANCER PATIENTS

Now fast forward to June 2007. Dr. Grutsch was crunching data, and it was looking good for the use of a test product with RNA fragments with the approximately 70 patients who had participated in the study.

Beljanski was right after all—these RNA fragments could accelerate the replacement of platelets in patients undergoing very aggressive therapy for cancer.

"The product was clearly helping the patients to maintain their platelet counts," Dr. Grutsch said. "This was a very exciting result. A natural product was helping our patients in a meaningful way to get through their chemotherapy. Many of these patients had failed several rounds of chemo-therapy—we had some patients with 10 or 11 uncompleted cycles—and high doses of these RNA fragments appeared to be helping these patients complete therapy on time and without a reduction in their doses. They had all sorts of cancer—breast, pancreatic, colon, lung. The thing they had in common was their chemotherapies were particularly aggressive—and with incredible failure rates. These were very challenging patients who had failed 9 or 10 earlier rounds."

This is such an important finding that Dr. Grutsch and the CTCA are anxious to begin enrolling patients in a larger clinical trial.

"Our next step is going to be to do a randomized clinical trial, which we hope will begin in January 2008. I think we are going to do some really important clinical trials now. The reason you do them right now is because if RNA therapy proves out in a larger randomized trial, it is a tool that will be important to cancer patients immediately.

"You really want to treat these people in a timely fashion, twice a month, and you could probably increase cure rates by a significant level. This could potentially be very important, and we want to be the first to discover it," he emphasized.

How difficult will it be to recruit patients? "Once our oncologists realize something potentially works, they are very good at recruiting all the patients; recruiting patients will not be an issue. You have to believe that the product has a real likelihood of working based on our first clinical trial. We are getting real experience with this product and feel really comfortable with it. But we have to keep going with more clinical trials, just as if we were working with an actual drug, because oncologists like lots of data points, as well they should. The things they do are challenging—just keeping patients alive from treatment cycle to treatment cycle. They have to know what they have to work with."

BUT, WHAT ARE RNA-FRAGMENTS?

As a biochemist, Dr. Beljanski knew that any cell, in order to duplicate, needs special and specific "primers" to catalyze the process of cell duplication. Besides the initial step of cell division, there is no other intention of these RNA fragments. All organisms function this way.

Dr. Beljanski prepared short fragments of RNA primers and found a natural way to extract purinerich nucleotides from Escherichia coli K12. (It must be noted that K12 is recognized by the National Institutes of Health as a totally innocuous E. coli strain.) These RNA fragments do not interfere with other cells. They simply support the body's ability to naturally enhance the generation of white blood cells and platelets.

"I think of the RNA fragments as food," said Dr. Grutsch, "a concentrated source of RNA. This product is food because RNA fragments can be essential nutrients. I know most people don't realize this. They're not up with the latest nutritional information. Every time you eat salads or meat, you are eating RNA, so your diet already has a large quantity of RNAs. But you get patients who are stressed, and if you give them the long-chain RNAs from this product, they actually maintain healthy platelet counts. We've tried other very similarly conceived ideas from other sources proclaiming to do the same thing, and they did not do it. There is some-thing about what Beljanski specifically uncovered that is completely unique.

"Our patients recovered faster. One of the biggest innovations is that the Food and Drug Administration now requires baby formula manufacturers to put long- and short-chain RNAs in their products too, so babies have less rounds of diarrhea. RNAs seem to be essential nutrients, especially if your body is under incredible physiological stress. But this information was really only uncovered in the last 10 to 15 years and, again, Beljanski provided so many of the research findings first and most accurately. Today, the data are overwhelming . In the last 10 years, of course, we have discovered that short-chain RNAs do all sorts of important things.

"Dr. Beljanski was 40 years ahead of his time. He spent his whole career trying to figure out what controls DNA replication. Part of this process is a small RNA molecule that has to exist for DNA replication to occur. However, while other researchers went on to different issues, Beljanski persisted in peering into the mysteries of life throughout his career."

Dr. Grutsch, nearly three decades removed from his blissful early days at the Pasteur Institute, has all the enthusiasm of the young scientist who thinks he can leave his mark on the scientific world thanks, of course, to the breakthrough work of Dr. Beljanski, a scientist who studied the very nature of life.

....

Resources

For more information about Dr. Beljanski's scientific research, please visit: www.beljanski.com

The Columbian Connection

By L. Stephen Coles, MD PhD

Excerpted with permission from HealthyLivinG Magazine
(HealthyLivinGMagazine.us)

Today, prostate cancer is the second most common cause of cancerous death among men worldwide, in particular throughout Europe and the United States. When prostatic tissue is examined microscopically, cancer is found in 50 per cent of males over age 70 and in virtually all males over age 90. Most of the time, such cancers never cause symptoms, but 3 percent of men exhibiting diseased prostate tissue changes die of the malignancy.

In fact, many men with prostate cancer now know it is probably not invasive and that they will die of other causes long before it ever spreads. Thus, extreme treatment isn't always the right way to go.

However even if it is not lethal, prostate cancer or enlargement can cause uncomfortable side effects that negatively impact a man's quality of life, such as problems urinating (i.e., a weak stream, getting up frequently at night, feeling the need to urinate but not actually doing so, etc.). These problems do not necessarily call for surgery but are too uncomfortable to ignore, and men in this situation need a less invasive solution.

One person who recognized this need is Columbia-based physician, Dr. Aaron Katz, a main stream urologist with a reputation as one of New York's leading prostate experts, according to *New York* magazine. Based at Columbia University, he is the director of the Center for Holistic Urology at the university's Physicians and Surgeons Hospital.

Dr. Katz was interested in research conducted by French molecular biologist Mirko Beljanski, Ph.D., (1923-1998) who spent over 25 years at the prestigious Pasteur Institute in Paris, France, studying DNA replication and transmission. Beljanski discovered that toxic molecules and carcinogens from the environment actually damage the physical structure of DNA, which he called DNA destabilization, leading to diseases such as cancer. He then looked for natural molecules that could help the body rid itself of the cells with damaged DNA while leaving the healthy cells unharmed. It was the molecules that Beljanski discovered, the plant extracts pao pereira and Rauwolfia vomitoria, that caught Dr. Katz's attention.

Dr. Katz met with Beljanski's daughter, Sylvie Beljanski, and his widow, Monique, who provided him with the background and explained the interest that was always shown by Beljanski in plants and treatments devoid of toxicity.

"I asked Sylvie a lot of questions about her father," he recalled. The two had several meetings at their New York City offices in which they discussed her father's work. She shared with Dr. Katz her father's many peer-reviewed scientific articles and research results, especially his applied research after leaving the Pasteur Institute.

Dr. Katz recalls, "I brought home a lot of reading material!" Bringing fresh eyes to Dr. Beljanski's research seemed to work. "I thought his science was excellent and definitely many decades ahead of his time. He was definitely the first to open up the whole field of structural DNA and in this alone his vision of the secrets of life was wholly unique and powerful.

"The next step was to take Beljanski's body of work and study it just as if it were any other pharmaceutical drug."

Everything had to be redone, he told Sylvie. American doctors want to see data from American labs. All the work Beljanski had done would have to be repeated in America and reconfirmed if it were to become accepted into the mainstream, and it would need to be extended into clinical trials. First Beljanski's basic findings pertaining to the plant extracts had to be tested again and confirmed in the Columbia University center's laboratory.

Dr. Katz had to start from the very beginning with the scientific team of his department, with cells in culture and then mice grafted with cancer cells.

Their research paid off big time with a notable peer-reviewed article in the November 2006 (29:1065-73) issue of the International Journal of Oncology that was titled, "Anti-prostate cancer activity of a beta-carboline alkaloid enriched extract from Rauwolfia vomitoria." Debra L. Bemis, Ph.D., and other top researchers from the Department of Urology College of Physicians and Surgeons, Columbia University Medical Center and the Center for Holistic Urology, reported on the anti-prostate cancer activity of this extract in vitro and in vivo.[1] In other words, the extract was significantly interfering with the progression of cancer much as Beljanski's own research had shown. Katz had done one of the most important things in science: he had independently confirmed another researcher's findings.

Indeed, Dr. Bemis went further and stated in an interview with the authors, "Our studies thus far indicate that both the rauwolfia and pao extracts suppress prostate tumor cell growth in culture, in vitro and also in vivo, but it appears to accomplish this effect through different mechanisms which we studied accurately." The data from the pao pereira studies was then published in the Journal of the Society for Integrative Oncology.[2]

"We found there was real scientific evidence that the combination of Rauwolfia vomitoria and pao pereira in a single dose, had a powerful inhibitory effect on the ability of prostate cells to grow and divide. That was very interesting to our team," said Katz.

A clinical trial began in 2006 and enrolled some 42 patients with elevated prostate specific antigen (PSA) readings (averaging 8 to 10 on the PSA scale) and a negative biopsy—a group of men that in the industrialized world numbers in the millions.

One of the primary goals of the clinical trial was to determine if the plant extracts were safe. The research team did a dose escalation trial. The trial started at two capsules but has gone much higher, and so far all doses tested have been without side effects.

"We now know that this combination of Beljanski's extracts can significantly lower PSAs in a 12-month period. Also we have had very few patients convert to prostate cancer and have found a number of patients who have had a dramatic improvement in their urinary symptoms. Men are clearly having less frequency, better streams and better flow rates. They are not getting up at night as often.

"The bottom line is that it appears our early results are reason to be very encouraged by Beljanski's extracts' ability to lower PSA and help older men urinate better, too."

So how important are Beljanski's findings to men's health? "There are a lot of men undergoing PSA screening," Dr. Katz said. "The PSA supposedly stands for 'prostate specific antigen' but I say it is more accurately 'patient stimulated anxiety.' When a man's PSA is elevated, there could be many reasons for this, having nothing to do with cancer. But what we know now is that these cells that are growing can develop into cancer, and we would like to stop them from doing so. Also if the cells keep growing even in benign fashion, they will grow around the urethra and push in on it and provoke urinary symptoms in men. That's where we want to lower the growth and division of prostate cells—and that's what we think we have shown with the extracts.

"Dr. Beljanski's fundamental vision has paid off in the way so many hoped for in his own lifetime. This compound has all of the molecular and biochemical studies showing why it works, how it actually recognizes the three-dimensional structure through the laddering and bonding of cancer DNA. He really did get it right," said Dr. Katz. "This is something that has great potential to help patients."

....

References

1. Bemis, D.L., el al. Anti-prostate cancer activity of a beta-carbo line alkaloid enriched extract from Rauwolfia vomitoria. Int J OnCol. 2006 Nov;29(5):1065-73.
2. Bemis DL, Capodice JL, Gorroochurn P, Katz AE, Buttyan R. Carboline alkaloid-enriched extract from the Amazonian rain forest tree Pao pereira suppresses prostate cancer cells. J Soc Int Oncol. 2009 Spring;7(2): 59-65.

How One Man's Courage is Helping Cancer Patients Across America

by David Steinman and L. Stephen Coles, MD, PhD

Excerpted with permission from HealthyLivinG Magazine (HealthyLivinGMagazine.us)

The history of science is filled with stories of men and women who, with their breakthrough discoveries, challenged the existing powerful interests of their day. These heroes of science (who often became political heroes as well) often demonstrated great courage to face off against extremely well-funded, established and profitable cartels like the intertwined interests of the chemical and food industries and the cancer and medical establishments. These scientific pioneers frequently suffered greatly for their courage in advocating truth over traditional theories, however unpopular and unwanted the truth may have been—at least by the most powerful moneyed interests.

Take, for example, Ignaz Philipp Semmelweis, born in 1818, an Austrian-Hungarian physician called the "savior of mothers." He discovered, by 1847, that the incidence of puerperal fever could be drastically reduced by implementing hand washing standards in obstetrical clinics. Puerperal fever (or childbed fever) was common in mid-19th century hospitals and often fatal, with mortality rates as high as 35 percent.

In 1847, as head of Vienna General Hospital's First Obstetrical Clinic, where doctors' wards had three times the mortality rates of those run by midwives, Semmelweis postulated that doctors who touched cadavers should wash with chlorinated lime solution prior to examining live patients. Despite his 1861 book which recounted statistically significant clinical trials where hand washing reduced mortality rates below one percent, Semmelweis' practice only earned widespread acceptance years after his death, when Louis Pasteur confirmed the germ theory.

In *The Secret History of the War on Cancer,* author Devra Lee Davis, Ph.D. tells how following World War II, the great industrial doctor and scientist Wilhelm Hueper discovered while working for Dupont that the benzidine dyes the company produced were causing occupational cancers. The company responded by suppressing his work and prohibiting him from ever visiting its industrial plants again. Hueper went to work for the recently formed National Cancer Institute where instead of being allowed to pursue his work, he was persecuted and branded as a communist, again because of the inordinate industry pressure from without and within the NCI.

Cancer prevention and treatment have become political because there is so much money at stake when it comes to protecting the profitable treatments that are sanctioned by the mainstream medical establishment and the commercial uses of toxic chemicals supplied by huge corporations. Like Semmelweis and Hueper, many scientists have been compelled to spread the news of their break through scientific discoveries for the public good, but the truth is often inconvenient, and sometimes the last thing society—and especially powerful petrochemical, medical, pharmaceutical, and agricultural interests—want to hear.

Yet history also shows that ultimately the truth wins out, and it is often a courageous few who protect the many.

A COURAGEOUS MOLECULAR BIOLOGIST IN FRANCE

Ironically, one such scientist, Mirko Beljanski (1923-1998), spent a quarter of a century performing much of his controversial research at the prestigious Pasteur Institute, the leading non-English speaking molecular biology institute in the world. Yet, although the Institutes own founders advocated the controversial findings of Semmelweis, in this case, Beljanski's work was strongly suppressed rather than supported. This is a story of courage and heroism worth telling.

Dr. Beljanski's key discoveries were that destabilized deoxyribonucleic acid (DNA) is a fundamental cause of cancer and that ribonucleic acid (RNA) can actually alter the master DNA blueprint. Today, his discoveries have become critical to developing selective nontoxic treatments for cancer, and to initiating an entirely new and important method of screening chemicals for toxicity. Beljanski's work with RNA fragments (as well as golden-leafed Ginkgo) have also led to an enormous breakthrough for support for cancer patients undergoing chemotherapy and radiation.

Beljanski's contributions in the field of cancer prevention and therapy, while known in his own time and appreciated by European doctors, immunology experts, and other clinicians, were particularly controversial in his beloved France, whose leading scientists at the Pasteur Institute were focused entirely on the mutational theory of cancer—and on winning the Nobel Prize! The story of Nobel Prize winner Jacques Monad and Beljanski, scientific rivals at the Pasteur Institute, is a classic.

Mirko's findings challenged France's prevalent orthodoxy of genetic research that was centered on the primacy of cellular DNA as the ultimate blue print of biological and genetic fate. Beljanski was a man who saw what others had only abstracted. He saw the three-dimensional changes to DNA structure. By his way of seeing DNA with spectrophotometry, he revealed the damaging effects of chemicals on the conformational structure of DNA before or without mutations in the genes. Beljanski's ability to interpret damage to the DNA double helix and assign meaning to what he saw in his scientific spectrophotometry (which was confirmed by the enhancement in DNA synthesis in vitro) represented a critical breakthrough in our understanding of cancer causation and treatment. Mutations in the DNA might only appear later, and by then it is often too late to reverse the damage.

Yet Beljanski's observations didn't fit into the scientific dogma of his day. Not only was he opposed by Monad, but the most dangerous attacks came from the French medical establishment after French President Francois Mitterrand successfully used the Beljanski formulas to prolong his own life in his battle with prostate cancer. Sadly for the rest of the world, once Mitterrand died, the French pharmaceutical and medical bureaucracy successfully attacked Beljanski mercilessly, suppressing his new discoveries for decades, and denying cancer patients potentially life-saving help. Most tragically, Beljanski was indicted in his beloved homeland and all of his scientific tools and writings were taken from his laboratory and destroyed. In America, of course, the Constitution guarantees a speedy trial and due process, but in France this slow torture of a scientist was condoned. Yet the European Court of Human Rights, when confronted with the evidence, later found that France had violated Beljanski's basic human rights. In Beljanski's case, in his adopted and beloved homeland of France, we have a shameful example of the harassment of a brilliant scientist who worked on behalf of the good of humanity.

In researching Beljanski's career, we became so absolutely troubled by what was done to him and the implications of his work—but we were also heartened by the greater receptivity to his findings here in the United States within our more liberalized health and medical system—and by the passion and determination of people who are dedicated to keeping Dr. Beljanski's flame burning brightly.

Despite the opposition he faced, Beljanski managed to publish more than 130 studies in peer reviewed scientific publications including those he authored with Nobel Prize winner Severo Ochoa. Beljanski's studies are being belatedly recognized as major contributions to the field of environmental medicine, particularly in cancer prevention and treatment and for innovative effective cancer support therapies (thanks to his RNA fragments).

The treatments based on Beljanski's molecules are being today used throughout Europe and North America by medical doctors and thousands of cancer patients: and, with more than one million Americans diagnosed with cancer each year, the number of patients who could potentially benefit from the Beljanski molecules is truly staggering. Beljanski's molecules could help millions of people globally to prevent and fight cancer. The public needs to know about Beljanski's research, particularly people who are dealing with cancer now.

Fortunately, the work of Beljanski is currently enjoying a renaissance because major institutions including Columbia University and the Cancer Treatment Centers of America have demonstrated the efficacy and mechanism of action of the Beljanski molecules. Now it Is time for their use to become the backbone of mainstream cancer treatment and for widespread acceptance of Beljanski's method of observing cellular damage to screen substances for carcinogenicity.

Indeed, Beljanski's findings are infiltrating into the mainstream cancer establishment that once persecuted or, even worse, ignored him. It is as if he is more alive now than ever. Beljanski's fundamental research and its dissemination may finally help the global health community win the war on cancer with improvements in prevention and treatment that truly offer a breakthrough that is desperately needed.

Beljanski's findings also offer a means of identifying a whole new class of chemicals that should be identified as early carcinogens, or what some experts refer to as pro-carcinogens or cancer promoters. These environmental chemicals cause cumulative damage to the cell's structural materials independent of genetic mutations. Indeed, it is as if genetic mutation tells only a small part of the story, as cellular interaction with these environmental chemical results in DNA destabilization, which in turn makes cells susceptible to uncontrolled proliferation (the definition of cancer). In other words, by using Beljanski's findings, we can identify toxic chemicals in the environment that set the stage for cancer, instead of simply waiting until the last minute ad primarily regulating only mutagens.

Today, scientists and medical doctors, particularly those from America and who espouse the use of integrative methods—also known as complementary and alternative medicine (CAM)—are embracing the Beljanski plant molecules, RNA fragments and his basic insights as integral to their primary cancer treatment support programs. Many people are surviving cancer that they probably would not have otherwise, and experiencing a better quality of life with the help of the Beljanski plant molecules and RNA fragments. This is a fact.

There is hope in the war against cancer. To seize a brighter future, however, it is imperative that everyone with cancer or a history of cancer or who is interested in prevention learn about the Beljanski plant molecules and RNA fragments.

....

Resources

For more information about Dr. Beljanski's scientific research, please visit: www.beljanski.com

---

Golden Leaf Ginkgo Extract for Radiation Protection and Skin Fibrosis

By L. Stephen Coles, MD, PhD
Excerpted with permission from HealthyLivinG Magazine
(HealthyLivinGMagazine.us)

The Ginkgo biloba tree is believed to be over 270 million years old. Individual trees may live as long as 1,000 years, growing to a height of 100 to 122 feet and with a trunk diameter of 3 to 4 feet. The tree is originally native to China and Japan, but has since been extensively cultivated throughout the world, thanks to its hardy nature. Although Asian cultures have used Ginkgo seeds medicinally for hundreds of years, the modern Western use of Ginkgo is limited exclusively to the leaf. The green leaves of the tree are usually harvested from trees growing in plantations in South Korea, Japan and France. But here, in this article, we only refer to a golden leaf Gingko extract, obtained according to a totally different mode of preparation, which confers a different type of activity.

The Ginkgo biloba tree is remarkably resistant to all kinds or pollution, viruses and fungi. For both biochemical reasons and because of its legendary resistance following the atomic bombings of Hiroshima and Nagasaki, it is one of the plants on which the late Dr. Mirko Beljanski chose to focus his attention. Thanks to a six-year contract with the French army, he was able to study protection against radiation. The contract included the study of an American agent for radiation protection called W2721, which offered an effective protection, but had to be administered intravenously and had to be kept at -4° F. (These constraints, not particularly compatible with the military's needs, were likely the reasons the product was later abandoned.)

As a result of his research contract with the French army, Beljanski was also able to witness the side effects of radiation firsthand. His contract allowed him to study several other substances besides W2721, and he went on to discover the protective effects of a special extract of Ginkgo biloba—the golden leaf Ginkgo biloba—different in its biochemical composition from all other greenleaf extracts of the plant. Sylvie Beljanski, daughter of the late Mirko Beljanski and President of Natural Source International, Ltd., explains: "The golden leaf Ginkgo biloba extract discovered by my father has very different properties than the green leaves we most commonly know, due to the time at which it is harvested and the unique extraction procedure he developed.1 Beljanski's extract is an excellent enzymatic regulator for radioprotection and for prevention of fibrosis. It also regulates immunoglobulin.

Medical descriptions of tumors resulting from radiation burns date back to 1828.2 Sirsat and Shrikhande reported that approximately 25 percent of burns cause tumors, and that the lowered immunity resulting from radiation and/or chemotherapy predisposes to malignant degeneration.[3][4]

J.W. Gofman, Professor Emeritus of Molecular and Cellular Biology at the University of California, Berkeley conducted a large-scale investigation involving scientists, doctors, etiologists and physicians. The investigation, entitled "Radiation from Medical Procedures in the Pathogenesis of Cancer and Ischemic Heart Disease" was published in November 1999. It states:

"Medical radiation, introduced as a treatment in 1896, is becoming a factor in approximately half of all fatal cases of cancer in the U.S. The proof cited in my 1999 monograph, which no one has refuted, indicated that approximately 250,000 people in the U.S. die prematurely each year from cancer and coronary diseases, with half the cases due to the unnecessary and excessive use of X-rays that they received over a lifetime.

"Radiation due to medical imaging is a necessary factor in approximately half of fatalities in the treatment of coronary diseases in the U.S." [5][6]

Dr. Beljanski demonstrated in several experiments that his original golden leaf ginkgo extract, through its normalizing effect on cellular enzymes, helps the tissues to remain in good health, even when they are exposed to extreme physiological stresses.[1]

Medical radiation induces burns and alters the action of ribonucleases (the enzymes which process RNA molecules). In a healthy cell, the normal function of these enzymes is to cleave RNAs and to provide cells the RNA primers they need to function. In some conditions of physical stress, these enzymes become deregulated, which can have a damaging effect on the health of cells and connective tissues. It is therefore critical to protect the skin from burns, whether from the sun or from ionizing radiation. [7][8]

Beljanski focused specifically on radiation-induced fibrosis, the scar tissue that forms as a result of exposure to ionizing radiation and that may take 6 to 12 months to develop. He demonstrated that skin cells exposed to radiation exhibit excessive RNase activity. However, when Beljanski added his special Ginkgo biloba extract, the excessive RNase activity was reversed. This golden leaf Ginkgo biloba preparation is an impressive example of a natural biological regulator that suppresses the pathological activity of RNase enzymes induced by radiation.

Although the mortality rate is low, suffering and subsequent complications from radiation-induced fibrosis are common. It is therefore important to protect the body during and several months following ionizing radiation treatments, due to the slow appearance of fibrosis. The late onset of pulmonary and cardiac effects is also a common side effect of ionizing radiation, which is, in turn, amplified by chemotherapy. [9][10]

The radiation-induced changes in nucleases are also linked to collagen production—a primary factor in the formation of scars. By restoring normal nuclease activity, Dr. Beljanski's researched Ginkgo biloba extract appears to normalize the development of scar tissue. When there are abnormally high amounts of gamma-globulins in certain inflammatory processes, this oral gingko extract use can aid a progressive return to normal values, with an immediate clinical amelioration.

Mirko Beljanski showed that his unique ginkgo preparation stimulated the in vitro synthesis of DNA from healthy skin, while at the same time inhibiting the synthesis of DNA isolated from mice melanoma.[1] The DNA synthesis being the first necessary event for cells' duplication explains the great benefits that one may observe while consuming Dr. Beljanski's gingko preparation: improved quality of skin and faster healing mechanism as showed in the results of a survey done on radiotherapy patients consuming the golden leaf Ginkgo biloba extracts.

Our skin's health and beauty is directly connected with its physiological state, and that, in turn, depends on the state of equilibrium in each of us.

The golden leaf Ginkgo plant extract prepared according to Mirko Beljanski's technique has been widely used in Europe for the last 20 years.

In particular, this Ginkgo extract has been combined with Pao pereira (Geissospermum) and Rauwolfia vomitoria extracts, two other plant extracts that Mirko Beljanski studied for the great benefit they may offer. Recent studies conducted at Columbia University Medical Center have extensively examined the mechanisms of action by which those two other extracts fight the proliferation of ab normal cells, with very interesting results.[11][12]

To that end, Sylvie Beljanski, who is well determined to continue her father's work as Head of Natural Source International Ltd. adds, "Continuing my father's research in the U.S. is of utmost importance in order to educate people about the amazing health benefits those plants can deliver to everyone. Today more than ever, with the recent dramatic worldwide events, creating awareness around this research has become crucial and everyone should be given the right answers on how to protect their health from environmental toxicity."

Learn more about Dr. Beljanski's scientific research at the following websites:

- www.beljanski.com which is the site for the Beljanski Foundation

- www.pubmed.com (to view Beljanski's studies and the recent paper from the International Journal of Oncology)

....

References

1. US Patent no. 5413787
2. Marjolin J.N.: Ulc- re. In: Adelon N.P. (Ed.): "Dictionnairede medicine," Vol. 21, 31-50, Bechel, Paris, 1828.
3. Sirsat, M.V., Shrikhande, S.S.: "Histochemical studies on squamous cell carcinomas or the skin arising in burn scars with special reference to histogenesis." Indian J. Cancer 3: 157-169, 1967.
4. Castillo and Goldsmith (1968) explained that lowered immunity in scar tissue predisposed the patient to malignant degeneration. Moreover, all burns alter tissue in the deoxyribonucleic acid at the cellular level, a product of mutations (Clairmont et al. 1979), themselves inducing new cancer.
5. Gofman, J.W. Preventing Breast Cancer. The Story of a Major, Proven, Preventable Cause of the Disease. ISBN 0932682960. Library of Congress Catalog Number LCCN 96-2453.
6. Gofman, J.W. Radiation from Medical Procedures in the Pathogenesis of Cancer and Ischemic Heart Disease: Dose-response studies with physicians per 100,000 population. ISBN 093268979. Library of Congress Catalog Number LCCN 99045096
7. M. Beljanski, "The Regulation of DNA Replication and Transcription. The Role of Trigger Molecules in Normal and Malignant Gene Expression." EVI Liberty (2003). (First Edition : Experimental Biology and Medicine, vol.8, Karger -1983), pp. 11-15
8. Causse, J.E., T Nawrocki, M. Beljanski, "Human Skin Fibrosis RNase Search for a Biological Inhibitor Regulator": Deut. Zeit. Fur Onk., 26, 5, 1994, pp. 137·139.
9. C. Nordau. M. Beljanski, "A Pioneer in Biomedicine," Evi Liberty Corp, New York, 2000, p. 118.
10. Rosen, I., Fischer, T. et al. "Correlation between Lung Fibrosis and Radiation Therapy Dose after Concurrent Radiation Therapy and Chemotherapy for Limited Small Cell Lung Cancer." Radiology 2001; 221:614.
11. D.L. Bemis, J.L. Capodice, et al. "Anti-prostate activity of a B-carboline alkaloid enriched extract from Rauwolfia vomitoria." Intern. J. of Oncology 2006, 29:1065

12. D.L. Bemis, J.L. Capodice. et al. "B-carboline alkaloid-enriched extract from the Amazonian rain forest tree Pao Pereira suppresses prostate cancer cells." J. of the Soc. for Integrative Oncology 2009. 7(2):59.

Prostabel Reduces Men's PSA Counts

Excerpted with permission from HealthyLivinG Magazine
(HealthyLivinGMagazine.us)

Aaron Katz, MD, is probably the most important clinician today when it comes to the fast-growing field of complementary medicine and men's health. Katz is also a national leader in cryosurgery, particularly focused on cryoablation. That his research is coming out of Columbia University, whose hospital and teaching schools are considered to be among the very best in the world, adds even greater credibility. He is also author of *Dr. Katz's Guide to Prostate Health* (Freedom Press, 2005).

In the case of Prostabel, Dr. Katz met with Sylvie Beljanski of Natural Source International, Ltd. Ms. Beljanski is the daughter of the late humanitarian and scientist Dr. Mirko Beljanski of the famed French Pasteur Institute and Monique Beljanski who was also a notable researcher and now lives in the United States.

The two had several meetings at their New York City offices in which they discussed Mirko Beljanski's work. Sylvie shared with Dr. Katz her father's many scientific articles and research results, especially his applied research after leaving the Pasteur Institute.

Dr. Katz recalls, "I brought home a lot of reading material!" Yet, bringing fresh eyes to Dr. Beljanski's research seemed to work. "I thought his science was excellent and definitely many decades ahead of his time. He was definitely the first to open up the whole field of structural DNA and in this alone his vision of the secrets of life was wholly unique and powerful."

With more than 130 peer-reviewed publications in his lifetime, Dr. Beljanski uncovered the secrets of the structure of DNA at the same time that others were trying to decipher the genetic codes of the double helix. Although genetic mutations became the buzzword of research for some four or five decades, these were largely one-dimensional ways of looking at the secret of life and could not account for earlier damage that occurred to the DNA before the presence of genetic mutations.

Beljanski's work is now becoming the basis for a whole new branch of research into the code of life. And it doesn't hurt that this research is showing promise in a major clinical trial at Columbia University.

STUDIED LIKE A PHARMACEUTICAL

Since that first meeting with Ms. Beljanski and her team, Dr. Katz, together with Columbia University, has gone on to develop scientific protocols to take Dr. Beljanski's body of work and study it for efficacy "just as if it were any other pharmaceutical drug."

"We went from cell cultures to laboratory experiments with animals and found there was real scientific evidence that the herbs [Rauwolfia vomitoria and Pao pereira] in Prostabel, when mixed together, had a powerful inhibitory effect on the ability of prostate cells to grow and to divide. That was very interesting to our team—and we wanted to go further and do clinical trials. I went back and spoke with Sylvie and I told her that there was no guarantee in any of this how things would turn out. "We don't know," I told her. "That's why we do these things. Natural Source International, Ltd. took a huge risk in going forward with our clinical trial because they know we are going to report the truth no matter what."

The clinical trial that Dr. Katz put together to study the health effects of Prostabel should interest all health-conscious men. Dr. Katz's team enrolled some 30 patients with elevated prostate specific antigen (PSA) readings (averaging 8 to 10 on the PSA scale) and a negative biopsy—a very interesting group that numbers in the hundreds of millions in the general population.

Millions of men have ticking time bombs in their prostates—they have elevated PSAs but they don't have cancer yet.

In some cases urologists prescribe Proscar (finasteride) to their patients, but this is a very powerful medical drug that has led to a number of side effects (depressed sexual libido, impotence, gynecomastia, and the potential for birth defects). In a world where medicine would be unbiased by profits, Proscar would not be considered a big hit because of these side effects. But it's what men nationwide are getting because it is one of the only drugs out there for this condition. And the idea for many men and their doctors of simply doing nothing ("watchful waiting") isn't an appealing alternative, either. After all, says Dr. Katz, "If you look at some of the clinical trials with men who have had a biopsy based on their PSAs—even men with PSAs of around 2 to 2.5 still have a 25 percent incidence of cancer. As you go above PSA readings of 10, some 70 percent of men are likely to develop cancer."

This is where Dr. Katz's work on Prostabel is so unique and powerful. From what the results show so far, Prostabel can produce favorable health benefits and give men the opportunity to do something positive to reduce their risk for more serious out-comes. Yet Prostabel has no side effects, is not a drug, and is well tolerated.

One of the goals of the clinical trial was to determine if Prostabel was safe. The research team did a dose escalation trial. They are about to en-roll their last patients at eight Prostabel capsules a day. The trial started at two capsules and so far all doses tested have been without side effects, said Dr. Katz.

"In addition, in this clinical trial, we are following them to look at quality of life issues and how the formula affects urinary function. At 12 months, everybody will have another biopsy. What do we know so far? As our researchers crunch numbers and prepare for our publications, I think there are some things we can safely say that we are seeing and that we can speak about generally.

"We now know that Prostabel can significantly lower PSAs in a 12-month period. Also, we have had very few patients convert to prostate cancer and have found a number of patients who have had a dramatic improvement in their urinary symptoms. Men are clearly having less frequency, better streams, and better flow rates. They are not getting up at night as often.

"All of this quite apparent improvement in their urinary flow and prostate problems has been an interesting finding for us. We simply did not expect to see so much help for enlarged prostates (since we're also examining the ability of the extracts to interact with cells at the DNA level). But I am very encouraged. We have even been going up to eight pills a day without adverse events. Nobody has dropped out of the trial from side effects, either, which shows a lot since you almost always have a few dropouts even on placebo.

"The bottom line is that it appears our early results are reason to be very encouraged by the ability of Prostabel to lower PSA and help men urinate better, too. In some way that we now realize, Prostabel may be better than saw palmetto, although we can't say for sure because we have not tested Prostabel against saw palmetto. Sure, we would love to do side-by-side comparisons with saw palmetto and finasteride."

In fact, Dr. Katz will be directing a new Phase 2 multicenter trial to answer additional questions about Prostabel on an even larger scale. Patients can begin enrolling now in the study by contacting the Center for Holistic Urology (see Resources).

SCIENCE OF PROSTATE HEALTH

So how important is Prostabel to men's health? "There are a lot of men undergoing PSA screening," Dr. Katz said. "The PSA supposedly stands for prostate specific antigen but I say it is more accurately patient stimulated anxiety. When men's PSA is elevated, there could be many reasons for this, having nothing to do with cancer.

"One of the more common reasons is that the prostate has grown in a benign fashion. The more prostate cells you have, the more PSA gets into your bloodstream. Still, because we don't know if it is benign or malignant, many men undergo a prostate biopsy to make sure they do not have prostate cancer. If it is negative, just benign growth, then doctors might prescribe finasteride or not do anything. But what we know now is that these cells that are growing can develop into cancer and we would like to stop them from growing into cancer. Also, if the cells keep growing even in benign fashion they will grow around the urethra and push in on it and provoke urinary symptoms in men.

"Many men in their 60s and 70s have this problem where their growth is benign but their stream is weak and they are getting up at night and don't urinate as well. That's where we want to lower the growth and division of prostate cells—and that's what we think we have shown with the extracts in Prostabel. That's why we do these trials: to learn about our medicines. After all, Viagra's use for erectile dysfunction was discovered after researchers were initially looking at lung conditions in men. We want to gather our data in a scientific system and sit back and look at the results and offer rational explanations and find the best way to use these tools in the interest of men's health."

ACCEPTANCE BY OTHER DOCTORS

Although American urologists have sometimes refused to take the European studies as seriously as those published in their medical journals, thanks to the pioneering work of Dr. Katz, Dr. Beljanski's work is gaining acceptance among colleagues— and more and more doctors are interested in how to integrate these natural remedies into their patient's health plans, says Dr. Katz, who is a popular medical conference speaker.

"We don't get any antagonism when we're working with our projects," says Dr. Katz. "What we're doing here at the Center for Urology at Columbia University is saying to people there may be a role for these compounds, and we are going to test them and we are going to put them through tough clinical testing, much as if they were a pharmaceutical, and see if they pass muster and see if they have a mechanism of action. Rather than just handing them out to patients, we are doing appropriate scientific investigations and testing them out in the laboratory and seeing how they work with the patients, and if you do that and if you run it through university settings, then you might be open to some criticism but much less. What we're seeing is helping patients.

"I met with the people at the company and they were very dedicated and they made the financial commitment to do the research. The technical fees, cell culture work—and now the clinical trial—none of this is without expense and, as I said from the start, we don't know what we will get. It says a lot for a company like Natural Source. Dr. Beljanski's fundamental vision of DNA has paid off in the way so many hoped for in his own lifetime. This compound has all of the genetic studies showing why it works, how it actually recognizes the three-dimensional structure through the laddering and bonding of cancer DNA. He really did get it right. This is something that has great potential to help patients."

Summary of the Research of Dr. Katz's Team

International Journal of Oncology (2006; 29:1065-73)

The tropical shrub, Rauwolfia vomitoria, is a medicinal plant used traditionally to treat a variety of ailments. A bioactive alkaloid, alstonine, present in this extract was previously shown to have anti-cancer activity against cancer cell lines. This study considers the potential anti-prostate cancer activity of this extract in vitro and in vivo.

Rauwolfia vomitoria extract standardized for alkaloid content was tested for ability to influence the growth and survival of the human LNCaP prostate cancer cell line. A WST-1 assay was used to measure cell growth, and cell cycle analyses were conducted with flow cytometry. Pathway specific microarray analyses were utilized to identify the effect of Rauwolfia extract on the expression of 225 genes. Mice xenografted with LNCaP cells were treated with the extract or placebo control, and tumor growth was measured for 5 weeks.

Rauwolfia extract decreased in vitro cell growth in a dose-dependent manner ($p < 0.001$) and induced the accumulation of G1 phase cells. PARP cleavage demonstrated that apoptosis was induced only at the highest concentration tested (500 µg/m) which was confirmed by detection of cells containing sub-genomic DNA. The expression of genes associated with DNA damage signaling pathway was up-regulated by Rauwolfia treatment, including that of GADD153 and MDG. The expression of a few cell cycle genes (p21, cyclin D1 and E2F1) was also modulated. Tumor volumes were decreased by 60%, 70% and 58% in the groups fed the 75, 37.5 or 7.5 mg/kg Rauwolfia, respectively (Kruskal-Wallis test, $p < 0.001$). The Rauwolfia vomitoria extract significantly suppressed the growth and cell cycle progression of LNCaP prostate cancer cells, in vitro and in vivo.

MESSAGE TO MEN BASED ON DR. KATZ'S RESEARCH

As more studies are published that confirm the results Dr. Katz is seeing with patients using Prostabel, men are seeking the product for both prevention and healthy cell protection as well as when confronted with more serious actual health problems.

The Prostabel formula combines Pao pereira and Rauwolfia vomitoria. What the research shows so far is that even at eight capsules daily there were no untoward side effects and nobody dropped out due to side effects.

Although the population of men who can benefit from Prostabel is much larger, the clinical trial focuses on men who have elevated PSAs and negative biopsies. These men might find that Prostabel inhibits overall cell growth and reduces their benign and malignant problems. Men are using Prostabel like saw palmetto, and Prostabel is now routinely used—for prevention and help with age-related prostate symptom—and it seems to be getting good results.

Prostabel is regulated as a dietary supplement in the United States and is not intended for the treatment, diagnosis or cure of a disease. To be sure, we also advise that any users think of it as a way to maintain the body's health, and that if appropriate, they work with a qualified health professional for serious conditions. Prostabel appears to initiate repair processes in the body at the DNA level, which leads to improvement in cellular health. Men with prostate cancer who use this formula should also use it only to support their health and what is working well, including the ability to initiate normal cellular repair processes. They should work with their primary care physician.

More and more men are turning to Prostabel. As a result, the company is being inundated with calls from doctors and patients alike. But the good news is the company is prepared to take these calls and provide the necessary information.

In addition, because the next study will be a multicenter investigation, men from throughout the United States will be eligible.

Men's Serious Prostate Health Support

Excerpted with permission from HealthyLivinG Magazine
(HealthyLivinGMagazine.us)

Directly inspired by Mirko Beljanski's 50 years of research in biochemistry and molecular biology, Prostabel® is an innovative and natural blend of Pao pereira and Rauwolfia vomitoria extracts that specifically promotes prostate cell health. Studies from Columbia University validate that Prostabel could be a breakthrough prostate health supplement—one adept at staving off men's most feared conditions.

In the November 2006 issue of the International Journal of Oncology, Debra L. Bemis, PhD, and Aaron Katz, MD, and other top researchers from the Department of Urology, College of Physicians and Surgeons, Columbia University Medical Center and the Center for Holistic Urology, reported on the anti-prostate cancer activity of the Rauwolfia vomitoria extract in vitro and in vivo. In this study, the extract was tested for its ability to prevent cell proliferation of the LNCaP prostate cancer cell line and to shrink LNCaP prostate tumors. In the case of both the Pao and Rauwolfia extracts, positive results on tumor shrinkage were observed. At the end of the experiment, tumors were removed and further analyzed, to determine if there was biochemical evidence that the extract induced apoptosis, an important and highly desirable healthy cell process by which damaged cells naturally end their replication process.

"Tumor volumes were decreased by 60%, 70% and 58% in the groups fed the 75, 37.5 or 7.5 mg/kg Rauwolfia, respectively," the researchers said. "The Rauwolfia vomitoria extract significantly suppressed the growth and cell cycle progression of LNCaP cells, in vitro and in vivo." At the highest levels, the Rauwolfia extract also caused apoptosis.

Indeed, the Columbia University researchers went further and stated, "Our studies thus far indicate that both the Rauwolfia and Pao extracts suppress prostate tumor cell growth in culture and in vivo, but appear to accomplish this effect through different mechanisms of action. We expect to publish our data from the Pao studies within the near future." In the meantime, different mechanisms of action for these two extracts mean chances are that the combination will be twice more effective against proliferation of unwanted cells.

This research builds on some 130 peer-reviewed articles Dr. Beljanski produced in his lifetime. Many of these studies illuminated for the first time that the DNA helix actually suffers structural damage and subsequently focused on the use of Beljanski's Oncotest to detail a botanical treasury of rare rainforest and other plants thought to aid in maintaining cell health.

The tropical shrub, Rauwolfia vomitoria, is a medicinal plant used traditionally to treat a variety of ailments. A bioactive beta-carboline alkaloid, alstonine, present in this extract, was previously shown by Beljanski to have anti-cancer activity against cancer cell lines. What's more, the Rauwolfia extract used for Prostabel has been purified of its reserpine content, another potent alkaloid used to treat high blood pressure but known to be toxic.

Many chemotherapy drugs today, like vinblastine and vincristine, are synthetic versions of natural plant molecules and they are modified for patentability, but because they are drugs, they can cause many side effects and are often extremely toxic.

However, the Beljanski extracts are far away from being drugs. They work far differently, have a different role, and they are not toxic. To begin with, the extracts are natural, not synthetic, and all of the active compounds they contain are natural as well. Prostabel utilizes the natural plants' molecules rather than synthetic, patented substances and is regulated in the U.S. as a dietary supplement. As such, it is explicit it will help by supporting and maintaining healthy cell processes.

Although specialists, including oncologists, and hospital integrative medicine programs are increasingly receptive and interested in offering alternative or complementary medicine or other modalities to their patients, these "complements," which might even include Prostabel, are thought of as supporting men's health and innately supporting the body's healthy responses. Often, Prostabel is recommended along with chemotherapy or radiation. It is not touted as a cure by any means. Perhaps this is why despite years of research in Europe on its extracts, Prostabel is one of the best-kept secrets in men's health.

One of Beljanski's long-term goals was to see his products used in conjunction with conventional therapies. He was sophisticated in this regard. Not only did he foresee the effectiveness of combining his extracts with mainstream chemotherapies, he generated data showing that these combinations were synergistic.

Prostabel is now the focus of a clinical trial at Columbia for men with elevated prostate-specific antigen (PSA); some 42 male subjects between 40 to 75 years of age who have an elevated PSA and a negative prostate biopsy within the past 6 months are being enrolled. Within one month of completing the study, the subjects will have a new prostate biopsy to assess change from the initial biopsy. All subjects will remain in the study for the 12-month duration. Nonetheless, in view of what he already knows, Dr. Katz, Director of the Center for Holistic Urology at Columbia, states of the Beljanski extracts, "They do have mechanisms of action and they can interfere with cell growth of prostate cancer."

HOW TO FIND PROSTABEL

Prostabel is available in the U.S. from Natural Source International. The company is working with health professionals to educate people about the Beljanski extracts. Fortunately, more and more doctors, including oncologists, are becoming interested in natural, scientifically supported formulas, such as Prostabel, and the interest will be even greater when the clinical trial results are published. For many men, the best time to act is now.

....

References

Bemis, D.L., et al. "Anti-prostate cancer activity of a beta-carboline alkaloid enriched extract from Rauwolfia vomitoria." Int J Oncol, 2006 Nov;29(5):1065-73.

Beljanski, M. "The anticancer agent PB-100, selectively active on malignant cell lines, even multidrug resistant." Genetics and Molecular Biology, 2000;23(1):29-33.

Beljanski, M. "Oncotest: a DNA assay system for the screening of carcinogenic substances." IRCS Medical Science, 1979;7:476.

Beljanski, M. & Beljanski, M.S. "Selective inhibition of in vitro synthesis of cancer DNA by alkaloids of B-carboline class." Expl. Cell. Biol., 50, 1982, pp.79-87.

Beljanski, M. & Beljanski, M.S. "Three alkoloids as selective destroyers of cancer cells in mice. Synergy with classic anti-cancer drugs." Oncology, 1986; 43:198-203.

....

Resources

If you are a consumer or health professional and have any questions or would like more information, contact Natural Source International at (888) 308-7066 (toll free) or (212) 308-7066. www.natural-source.com

Prostabel is currently the focus of a clinical trial at the Columbia University Center for Holistic Urology for men with elevated PSA. This clinical trial is currently open. For more information call Dr. Geovanni Espinosa at 212-305-3790 or e-mail him at ge2108@columbia.edu.

Learn more about Dr. Beljanski's scientific research at the following websites:

- www.beljanski.com (this is the CIRIS site known in French as the Scientific Center for Information, Research and Innovation)

- www.mbschachter.com

- www.pubmed.com (to view Beljanski's studies and the recent paper from the International Journal of Oncology).

- www.self-helpcancer.org

- To find a doctor who can help you to use the Beljanski plant extracts in your program, visit the American College for Advancement of Medicine website at www.acam.org and use their physician referral service.

DR. BELJANSKI—SCIENTIST, HUMANITARIAN

Molecular biologist Mirko Beljanski, PhD (1923–1998), in association with his wife and research associate, Monique, conducted research into the respective roles of DNA and RNA in the development and cure of cancer, first at the Pasteur Institute in France (1948-1978) and then at the Faculty of Pharmacy at Chatenay Malabry (1978-1988), according to an Internet information site (www.self-helpcancer.org).

According to the site, "Beljanski's primary thesis is that cancer is caused not only by DNA mutations, but also by damage to the hydrogen bonds that hold the two strands of the DNA double helix together."

Beljanski's work, which is of vital importance to the science of cancer prevention and therapeutics, helps explain, for example, "why an excess of certain hormones such as estrogen and testosterone (and other steroids, too) is carcinogenic, although they do not appear to be the direct cause of mutations."

Beljanski also developed a test to determine which substances could destabilize DNA function, leading to cancerous cell proliferation, and conversely, which kind of substances could repair or cause programmed death (apoptosis) of damaged and cancer-forming DNA. "Among such molecules, he discovered, are the naturally occurring plant alkaloids alstonine, flavopereirine, serpentine and sempervirine, which are able to distinguish between normal and cancer-forming DNA causing the death of the malignant cells (apoptosis or cell cycle arrest). Beljanski conducted many trials on the anti-cancer properties of these substances. He was able, for example, to cure an appreciable proportion of mice with lymphoma. Other in vitro studies showed that his Pao pereira extract was active against a number of other cancer cell lines (brain, breast, ovarian, prostate, kidney, thyroid, pancreatic, colon, liver, skin), including those that were multidrug resistant."

During his 10 years at CIRIS (Scientific Center for Information, Research and Innovation), he demonstrated that his substances also work in synergy with radiation or standard chemotherapy agents, providing better results than with the chemotherapy alone.

In his lifetime, Dr. Beljanski authored two books. *The Regulation of DNA Replication and Transcription* is available in English, while *La Santé Confisquée* is available in French.

High PSA, Negative Biopsy, Now What?

by L. Stephen Coles, MD, PhD
Excerpted with permission from HealthyLivinG Magazine
(HealthyLivinGMagazine.us)

So your prostate-specific antigen (PSA) reading is higher than you'd like, perhaps even rising suspiciously, and your urologist has ordered a biopsy, which proved negative. Now it is time to breathe a sigh of relief—and to get a reality check.

93

WHAT TO DO NEXT?

Well, first of all, you are not alone. Every older man is aware of prostate health issues. The prostate plays a major role in men's health, including affecting his urinary flow, sexual function, enjoyment of life and ability to travel. But today, unfortunately, millions of men have experienced similar prostate problems.

What is the PSA anyway? According to PSA Rising, a cancer survivors' group, "The PSA test is a simple blood test to measure how much PSA a man has in his bloodstream at a given time The PSA test is the most effective test currently available for the early detection of prostate cancer. Since the PSA test came into use in the United States, the death rate for prostate cancer has fallen by one-third In 2005. A Harvard study found that men who have yearly PSA tests are nearly three times less likely to die from prostate cancer than those who don't have annual screenings. The University of Pittsburg Cancer Institute says PSA testing and digital rectal examination (DRE) 'are crucial in detecting prostate cancer in its early stages. when it usually produces no physical symptoms.' PSA testing is also used to monitor the progress of prostate cancer that has already been diagnosed."

As many men know, an elevated or rising PSA can signal potential problems down the road. Suspicious cells can become rogue. That's why your urologist could recommend frequent biopsies.

But on the other hand, extreme treatment isn't always the right way to go. Even in recent times it has not been uncommon for men treated with radiation to experience secondary cancers. Yet, we also know that dietary changes, including more flaxseed for example, exercise and use of specific herb combinations can provide great health support.

This might be a good lime to support your prostate health and use an effective herbal support formula.

Researchers writing in The Journal of Urology (2002,168;6 2505-09) say, "Complementary therapies are used by a large number of patients."

In a study in the November 2003 issue of Urology , researchers noted that in their study of prostate health patients, "Almost one-third (29.8 percent) reported using complementary and alternative medicine (CAM)."

THE RESEARCHER WHO DISCOVERED HOW PLANTS BENEFIT MEN'S HEALTH

Molecular biologist Mirko Beljanski, PhD may well have discovered the answer to a negative biopsy with rising PSA during 25 years of research at the Pasteur institute in Paris, France, one of the most prestigious laboratories in the world. During his research he discovered two plant extracts, Pao pereira and Rauwolfia vomitoria, that act at the cellular level to help the body rid itself of damaged cells. Beljanski published some 133 peer-reviewed articles over his lifetime, including those that demonstrated the profound benefits to cellular DNA that could be obtained with ingestion of the plant extracts. His formulas have become available in the United States and their use for just such conditions is likely to grow as result of a recently published study—and as preliminary results become known of a just-completed clinical trial on these two extracts conducted at Columbia University's Physicians and Surgeons Hospital.

THE NEW YORK DOCTOR WHO PIONEERED THEIR USE

Dr. Aaron Katz, one of New York's leading urological surgeons according to *New York* magazine, recently conducted a series of studies and a clinical trial at the Columbia University Center for Holistic Urology looking al Beljanski's two extracts. Dr Katz is director of the center, which is based at the Physicians and Surgeons Hospital al Columbia.

"Initially, I learned about Beljanski's extracts from my patients who were taking them for prostate conditions and using them for effectively lowering their PSAs," said Dr Katz, "and it wasn't just one patient; it was a lot of patients. So I said you know what? Maybe there's something to this. Maybe this is real."

Dr Katz recalls, "[Beljanski's] science was excellent and definitely many decades ahead of his time. He was definitely the first to open up the whole field of structural DNA and in this alone, his vision of the secrets of life, was wholly unique and powerful. The next step was to take Beljanski's body of work and study it clinically."

The Columbia team's preclinical findings were published this year in the Spring 2009 issue of the Journal of the Society for Integrative Oncology (7,2 59-65). Dr. Debra Bemis and co-researchers from the Center for Holistic Urology reported that, "Bark extracts from the Amazonian rainforest tree,

Geissospermum vellosii (Pao pereira), enriched in beta-carboline alkaloids, have significant anticancer activities in certain preclinical models. Because of the predominance of prostate cancer as a cause of cancer-related morbidity and mortality for men of Western countries, we preclinically tested the in vitro and in vivo effects of a Pao pereira extract against a prototypical human prostate cancer cell line, LNCaP. When added to cultured LNCaP cells, Pao pereira extract significantly suppressed cell growth in a dose-dependent fashion and induced apoptosis."

This study, of course, comes on the heels of another study published in the November 2006 issue of the International Journal of Oncology (29;5 1065-73) regarding the Rauwolfia vomitoria extract. Again, Dr. Bemis and other top researchers reported on the highly beneficial inhibition exhibited in vitro and in vivo.

These results led the Center for Holistic Urology at Physicians & Surgeons Hospital to conduct a recently completed clinical trial.

The clinical trial, which began in 2006, enrolled some 42 patients with elevated PSAs (averaging 8 to 10 on the PSA scale) and a negative biopsy—a group of men that numbers in the millions worldwide. Dr Katz looked at quality of life issues and how the formula affects urinary function. Hopefully, final findings will be available soon, since Dr. Katz has informed me that the study is completed with all results. Here is what we do know: "I think there are some things we can safely say that we are seeing and that we can speak about generally," says Dr. Katz. "We now know that this combination of Beljanski's extracts (Prostabel®) can significantly lower PSAs in a twelve-month period. Also, we found a number of patients who have had a dramatic improvement in their urinary symptoms. Men are clearly having less frequency, better streams and belier flow rates. They are not getting up as often during the night.

"All of this quite apparent improvement in their urinary flow and prostate problems has been an interesting finding for us. We simply did not expect to see so much help for enlarged prostates (since we're also examining the ability of the extracts to interact with cells at the DNA level). But I am very encouraged. We have even been going up to eight pills a day without adverse events. Nobody has dropped out of the trial from side effects either, which shows a lot since you almost always have a few dropouts even on placebo."

So how important are Beljanski's findings to men's health? "There are a lot of men undergoing PSA screening," Dr. Katz said. "The PSA supposedly stands for prostate specific antigen, but I say it is more accurately, 'patient stimulated anxiety.' When men's PSA is elevated, there could be many reasons for this, having nothing to do with cancer. One of the more common reasons is that the prostate has grown in a benign fashion. The more prostate cells you have, the more PSA that gets into your bloodstream."

In this case, men have a very viable option to help support their health and do something positive. They should definitely work with their doctor, improve their diet, add flaxseed, for example, and omega-3 fatty acids, but I would urge a serious look at these two extracts, particularly in just such situations. This combination offers real benefits, based on real science.

A Story Told By An ARVN Soldier

The Need for a Formulation of a Just Cause for the ARVN
Chinh Nghia QLVCH (m)
http://www.patriotfiles.com/archive/generalhieu/chinhnghia_arvn-2.htm
Reprinted with Permission

Lacking objectivity and an analysis-synthesis of scientific method, the majority of foreign news media and historians have mistakenly assessed the ARVN as merely an army at the service of the policy of French colonialism and subsequently of the American policy in Vietnam, in the internationally strategic point of view, while ignoring the reality aspect and the ideological evolution of the ARVN as well as the everchanging historical facts. People with academic diplomas and the superb news media system of the free world have misguided the average mind of the general public, and of outer layer of the academic intelligentsia as well. The North Vietnamese Communists, on the other hand, have used such skewed assessments as a legalistic justification for the imprisonment and torture of hundreds of thousands of military and political personnel of the Republic of Vietnam after their invasion of South Vietnam, and for the death of a multitude of innocent Vietnamese who perished in the waters and in the hands of pirates while attempting to escape by sea in search of freedom. Fortunately, the free world, including the United States, had shown compassionate responsibility in welcoming the victims of the Communist regime.

Recently, the phenomenon of South Vietnamese flags fluttering in the skies all over the free world, the funeral ceremony for a couple of ARVN soldiers conducted by the US Army in Arlington cemetery, the erection of memorial sites in the honor of American and Vietnamese combatants, and conferences and symposiums on the role and just cause of the ARVN, are starting points leading toward an official and legal tribute which will be paid to the ARVN in the very near future. The consequence of such tribute is that the surviving ARVN will have the legal justification to liberate the entire Vietnam or to lend support to a revolution by the people within the country, which will eradicate the dictatorship of the Communist Party in the future in principle, although the ARVN has ceased to exist in reality. Furthermore, out of sense of responsibility, the free world will back up the surviving ARVN in its effort to restore freedom in Vietnam because they had abandoned their ally in 1975. In addition, in the world's opinion, the Communists will become war criminals for their acts of imprisonment and torture or massacre of prisoners.

Rendering honor to the ARVN in the future can be misconstrued or criticized by the communist bloc as merely a shortterm policy of the free world. Therefore, paying tribute to the just cause of the ARVN must be demonstrated and evaluated objectively by historians of the world. This story told by an ARVN soldier does not have the ambition of proving this premise, but only the wish of providing genuine and living facts related to this premise.

Historians will find thousands of similar stories during these past three decades, which will allow them to analyze and synthesize objectively and scientifically for a just cause premise of the ARVN. These are the conditions for the just cause to attain transparency and magnanimity in the future. Furthermore, memoirs of communist cadres, declassified American, Chinese and Russian documents from various archives, and current movements reclaiming freedom and democracy by Vietnamese inside the nation are valuable treasures for historians to compare and to evaluate the just cause of the ARVN.

ASPIRANT LIEUTENANT BUI THUONG

I had the honor of knowing Aspirant Lieutenant Bui Thuong when he was assigned as executive officer of the recon company belonging to 46th Infantry Regiment around September 1963.

He once was a Catholic monk; he enlisted in the army in order for his children and his people to enjoy the freedom of religion not to become a slave to the French after he heard the news that the Communists in Quang Binh Province killed his father because of his Catholic belief. During his military service in the French army, he witnessed the difference in convictions among the Vietnamese soldiers: some joined the army because of economic reasons or to become servants to the French; some, like him, joined the Communists to fight against the French out of patriotism, but then left the Communists because they refused to join the Communist Party; some, realizing that Communism was at odds with the Vietnamese cultural heritage, chose to lean on the French power to fight against the Communists at the initial stage, with the intention to reclaim national sovereignty once they matured politically and militarily. After 1950, he noticed that the majority of the military personnel preferred nationalism to slavery under the French. By 1965, he saw that the ARVN had transformed entirely, from a composite army in terms of ideology to an ARVN with a strong aspiration of national independence. He quit the Can Lao party, took leave of his wife and six children and volunteered for a combat unit, the 46th Infantry Regiment in September 1963, but he never revealed the motive behind his action. Besides longrange reconnaissance tasks in Hau Nghia Sector, the Recon Company/46th Infantry also assumed the task of building strategic hamlets, which provided him with ample opportunities of exercising his patriotism, his leadership, and his skills in mass propaganda. He often visited and chatted with soldiers, and nurtured their patriotism by explaining to them the just cause of the ARVN. In particular his performance in the area of mass propaganda was quite inspirational to me. He often organized political sessions geared to the simple minds of the villagers, with great attention paid to the seating protocol: the presiding role was always given to the head of the village who sat at the first row among the elders; the next rows were assigned to the younger audience; and the last rows were reserved to the Recon Co/46th Infantry. He did not lecture much, but rather focused on listening to the wishes and questions of the villagers. His answers reflected his political convictions that the Nation takes precedent to Religions, and Religions should not interfere with politics; all Religions should be treated equally; freedom of religion is a legal entity in the RVN constitution; the Army assumes the task of defending the territories of a free Vietnam and protecting the South Vietnamese people against the threat or massacre of the Communists; South Vietnam does not accept the general referendum as dictated by the Geneva Accord, because President Ngo Dinh Diem did not participate in and did not sign this accord; and the RVN is a legal government elected by the people after the Geneva Accord, championing freedom and democracy; the Communist regime in the North is an unconstitutional regime because the North has never organized a free election to select Communism over freedom and democracy, or elect Ho Chi Minh to be the leader in the North; the Communists tricked the Vietnamese into opposing the French in order to save the country, because in reality the Communist party was an instrument in the expansion of Communism, lead by Communist Russia and China...

After more than a month building strategic hamlets, the recon company returned to its independent longrange recon role. The affection shown by the villagers in the farewell ceremony, the decreasing of deserters down to zero, while the number of VC killed or captured increased within a month were proofs of Aspirant Lieutenant Bui Thuong's exceptional leadership and charisma among the population.

He once again demonstrated his combat experiences, his courage, and his compassion during the period the company conducted longrange recon independently. He always volunteered to go with the lead platoon in order to share his combat experiences with the young platoon leaders. Every time he saw soldiers and me clapping our hands in delight when artillery shells hit bull eyes he looked at us with an air of concern and reservation. He was not sure the enemy got killed and worried those innocent villagers and animals got hurt. When nighttime came he started arguing those artillery shelling could harm the just cause of the ARVN, because he had witnessed indiscriminate artillery shelling on innocent peasants and piracy acts committed by the French army. If there was definitely no indications of the enemy being hit by artillery shells that night, he would lecture me on sensitivity toward innocent peasants then he would reprimand me for my tendency of showing off my skill in the use of artillery. Such nights reminded me of bedtime lectures I received from my mother for all of my daytime vagaries with other kids who were my friends. During his lecture, I fell asleep and started snoring. Next morning, as soon as I opened my eyes, he resumed his lecturing for falling asleep while he had not finished pouring out his inner thoughts. Upon seeing my laughing out loud, he burst out laughing louder than me, because it suddenly dawned onto him that my infantlike face reminded him of his children's faces during the time he lived in Saigon: they also fell asleep like me each time he lectured them at bedtime. He suddenly changed his facial expression into seriousness and defended me in saying that by using pre emptive artillery fire could limit casualties before the company assaulted, especially since the reconnaissance company was operating independently and therefore it needed artillery and air supports to cover and encourage the combatants. And so, no matter what he said, he found a way to justify it! He kept on lecturing and I kept on doing it my way!

During a longrange recon operation along River Vam Co Dong, the Recon Company did not encounter enemy resistance while maneuvering the whole morning. Aspirant Lieutenant Thuong suspected that the enemy would ambush the last planned target; he cautiously deployed his unit in an open space on crouching positions before launching the lead platoon to assault the dense forest. Following an hour of continuous artillery pounding this last objective, the Recon Company assaulted the edge of the forest after crossing the open space of the rice paddy without encountering any enemy resistance; however, he started to grunt upon seeing two dead cows hit by artillery fire lying at the edge of the forest; he kept on grilling me how to compensate the poor owners of these two cows; then he scolded me for calling in concentrated artillery firepower. Suddenly his facial expression changed rapidly, from sadness to sternness of a martial arts master, when two soldiers showed him a weapon stained with an enemy's fresh blood. He quickened his steps, moving forward with his lead platoon in the pursuit of the fleeing enemy that had been heavily decimated by our artillery firepower. Once again I witnessed with surprise the transformation of his facial expression, from fiery as of a warrior to benevolent as of a saint, when he saw an enemy deadly wounded by our artillery fire. He gave order to the medic to treat the prisoner's head wound, who was left behind by his comrades, then he knelt down next to him and asked him what could he possibly do at his very last moment. Just a few drops of water had allowed the wounded enemy to depart life in comfort and in peace, following a long sigh. He hastily closed the enemy's eyelids and said a prayer of deliverance for him. This was the first time the soldiers witnessed the sainthood trait of him. That night he asked me out of curiosity why I did not pray Buddha for the enemy because he knew I was a Buddhist from Hue.

A few weeks later, the Recon Company operated at regimental level in order to penetrate deeply into a VC stronghold near to the Cambodian border in Duc Hue District. A friendly battalion fell into an ambush and clashed heavily with the enemy at the last objective. Orders came from the Command Post of 46th Infantry to attack the rear of the enemy from the left flank of the friendly battalion; Aspirant Lieutenant Thuong volunteered to accompany the two lead platoons with me because he well knew I was eager to come to the rescue of a classmate, Vo Tinh, who was wounded while commanding his company's counterattack. At that moment, foes and friends were too close to one another, rendering the use of artillery impractical. Aspirant Lieutenant Thuong and I, together with the two platoons gave assault into the enemy line after throwing diversionary smoke grenades. Seeing me lurching forward with a tiny pistol, he managed to run before me with an automatic rifle to give me cover. The enemy, who was within 10 meters, gunned him down. Two grenades thrown by the soldier on my left cut down four enemies, allowing me to kneel down next to him. He passed away so fast, without pain; his eyes remaining wide open as if he wanted to keep looking at the enemy. I closed his eyelids and held his body and cried uncontrollably like a child. Dear Thuong, why did you have to die while the country needs you more than me! You closed the enemy's eyelids, but the enemy did not do the same to you! You prayed for the enemy, but the enemy did not pray for you! As for me, I dare not pray Buddha for you because I know you are a Catholic saint.

CORPORAL TRAN TAN

I had the honor of knowing Corporal Tran Tan when he was assigned to the 2nd Company of 1/8th Battalion as a 2nd private. Seeing he was rather frail, I appointed him a cook in the Headquarters Headquarters Company. He was disappointed with this assignment and requested to be transferred to the recon squad of 2nd Company. I turned down his request because this unit was established outside the table of organization and equipment of an infantry company, and was composed of volunteers with ample combat experiences. After two weeks, he had demonstrated his cooking talents, and started seeking to converse with me because we had the same Hue accent. He opened up by talking about his family situation: his father was killed by the VC because he had joined the Dai Viet party to oppose the French and even the VC; he was also a member of Dai Viet, and had to leave his paternal village and took refuge at a relative's home in Hue's inner city; still, Hue was too small in allowing him to blend in, which compelled him to take his wife and two children to Saigon; in July 1964, seeing that the military situation had worsened seriously, he decided to join the army to help the country. He used to observe the recon squad practicing hand combat with me every day, and one day he took the courage to challenge me when I was practicing hand combat with the squad leader. To my surprise, he countered all my attack moves with ease and dexterity.

Then, with lightning speed, he closed in behind me and locked my body. I attempted to unlock his grip, but all my efforts failed. Suddenly, he loosened up his locking position and allowed me to regain the upper hand with an elementary counter move. Soldiers clapped their hands to congratulate me, unaware of my embarrassment while I was standing in front of a true martial arts master. I bowed to him and considered him my teacher in martial arts. While the soldiers were startled by my deference toward him, he modestly requested to become a member of the recon squad. From that moment on, he became a longrange scout and the hand combat instructor of the recon squad. He used to put a ginger candy into my hand whenever I joined the recon squad in night ambush outings. The taste of mild sugar flavor mixed with hot ginger flavor kept my mind alert while waiting for the enemy to show up.

Each such time, I heard the chucklings of the longrange scouts lying nearby me; they spread the rumor that Tan tried to bribe me with ginger candies to make me accompany the recon squad. In reality, Tan did the same favor to them when he saw they too were tired or bickering with one another. From that moment on he got the nickname of the "candy long range scout". The word "keo" in Vietnamese means "stingy", and it suited him because he did not drink or gamble and was very stingy in his personal expenses. His wife always received in full all of his paychecks, except when he needed to buy ginger to mix with sugar that was part of his monthly ration.

I retain an unforgettable anecdote when the recon company operated in Tan Thanh Dong belonging to Binh Duong Sector. One evening, he asked me if I wanted to catch a VC fundraising operator that night or not. I was surprised and asked him about this intelligence information. I learned that he had set up an intelligence network among the local people three weeks after we started to operate in this area. Not convinced, I nevertheless decided to accompany the intelligence squad. Tan led the squad and I followed his footsteps in the night. The intelligence squad crawled through the door of a house with lights still on. I saw the fundraising operator sitting comfortably at a desk, counting the money. I plunged in to catch him alive, when I heard a burst of bullets rushing by me toward the direction of the kitchen. I realized that it was the quick thinking minded Dai Viet member, private Tan, who had saved my life when I saw two enemies' corpses with two automatic rifles lying on the floor. He was promoted to corporal in this raid.

On May 8, 1965, 1/8th Battalion was attached to 9th Regiment in operation Loi Phong in the VC stronghold of An Nhon Tay. The entire 9th Regiment and 1/8th Battalion fell into the enemy's ambush by 1:00 p.m. Both units fought valiantly and repulsed several assaults until ammunition ran out; however, there were no artillery and air supports for three hours. Finally, the regimental commander had to order his troops to withdraw to the nearby empty rice paddies in order to maneuver toward Cu Chi district of Hau Nghia province. 1/8th Battalion covered the rear and 2nd Company covered 1/8th Battalion's rear in this troop retreat without air and artillery supports. The enemy knew our intention to withdraw and kept on assaulting 1/8th Battalion and fired heavily at the combatants of the battalions of 9th Regiment who were running uncovered in the rice paddies. I witnessed hundreds soldiers with yellow scarves around the neck gunned down all over the rice paddies, then those with red scarves around the neck of the two companies and the HHC of Captain Cua in the hundreds while 2nd Company was repulsing two enemy's assaults to cover Captain Cua's retreat. I witnessed Tan killing many enemies with bayonet and bare hands in the last close combat, before the company attempted to catch up with 1/8th Bn HHC because Captain Cua lost control of his two companies that were running ahead of him. When the recon squad pierced enemy's encirclement line to escape to the open rice paddies, nobody had munitions left to lend cover fire for the rear troops, Tan had the initiative to crawl to a machine gun of a yellowscarfed gunner dead long time ago, and used it to fire at the enemy in pursuit of the last units of 2nd Company. At that moment four helicopters appeared unexpectedly and circled above the target to support the last troop units that just broke out of enemy's encirclement and poured out into the open rice paddies. He abandoned the machine gun, which ran out of bullets with its canon still hot red and ran toward the back. He immediately seized a light machine gun from a yellowscarfed soldier KIA and fired directly at about 30 enemies who just emerged from the edge of the forest. I witnessed a multitude of enemies gunned down when he still had two bullet clips in his hands. Suddenly I saw Tan collapse with the light machine gun. I crawled quickly toward him and grabbed his hand right at the moment he exhaled his last breath. I closed his eyelids and let 4 long-range scouts took turn to carry his body along with the company to catch up with Captain Cua who was waiting. The Captain embraced me and we wept together in sorrow for the lost of a beloved soldier KIA. Up in heaven, Corporal Tran Tan no doubt knew that he was the only one among all the soldiers who participated in this operation whose body was carried to Cu Chi district that night, because the 2nd Company and one battalion of the 9th Regiment had to stay behind in order to follow the rescue troops in the task to gathering dead bodies of friendly troops the next day.

Two days later, I visited the families of KIA soldiers at the quarters of soldiers' families in the base camp after I left General Tran Thanh Phong's office. Tan's wife and two children donned in funeral white dresses were mourning next to his coffin in a room covered by incense burning. I knelt in front of him with incense sticks in hands to pay tribute to a talented martial arts master, a patriotic member of Dai Viet party and a valiant combatant of the ARVN. I respectfully handed to Tan's wife his wallet and an envelope containing collection money from members of 2nd Company. She held the wallet to her chest as the last gift he reserved for her, and then she burst into tears, "My love! Why have you departed while we have not yet fulfilled our dreams!? Rest in peace, I will do my best to raise dutifully our children."

I don't know the whereabouts of Tan's wife and his two children; have they grown up to become good citizens? Are they allowed to embrace the party of their liking or have they been indoctrinated with communism? Do they know and are proud that they had a hero of the ARVN as a father? As for me, each year on May 8, I burn incense sticks with a ginger candy to commemorate the one who had saved my life, a martial arts master and a fearless combatant of the ARVN.

COLONEL NGUYEN VAN CUA

I had the honor of knowing Colonel Nguyen Van Cua when he became 1/8th Battalion Commander with the rank of captain. He demonstrated the gallantry of an elder classmate when he came to my defense appearing before an authoritarian division commander. When troops of 2nd Company just jumped out of trucks in the 5th Infantry Division's parking lot on May 10, Captain Cua and two company commanders in impeccable uniforms signaled me to follow them to report to the division commander. Upon entering the office I noticed immediately that the pair of two barn owl like eyes of Brigadier General Tran Thanh Phong were staring at my dirty and blood stained outfits. He suddenly banged the desk in anger, "What type of officer dresses like a beggar!" I was still affected by the heroic deaths of Tan and combatants of my company, and went for broke, criticizing the division commander for delaying air and artillery supports and munitions supplies as well for his absence on the battlefield. He tore the dossier that contained an award proposition to the 1/8th Battalion, and then rang the bell to call in the military policemen to imprison me. Captain Cua calmly stood up and requested to be imprisoned with me, and then the two company leaders also requested the same treatment as the battalion commander. When Captain Hoang, Class 15/VNMA, let in two military policemen, Captain Cua had just finished recounting the battle occurring at An Nhon Tay. General Phong dismissed the two MPs then apologized for his out of line tantrum.

A few days later, Captain Cua came to have dinner with me and slept over with the 2nd Company. That night, he confided in me his patriotic ideal, his revulsion of the massacre of patriots who fought against the French and the communist inhumane killing of Cao Dai's and Hoa Hao's religious leaders because they did not embrace communism; he foresaw the threat of communism and decided to join the army to fight against the communists, then the French, in order to regain independence for Vietnam.

Around two weeks later, 2nd Company got the chance to revenge the deaths of Tan and other combatants of 2nd Company in the battle of An Nhon Tay. In the road clearing operation along QL 13 from Bung Cau to Ben Cat of Binh Duong province, the entire 1/8th Battalion minus 2nd Company fell into the ambush of an enemy's battalion. 3rd Company was ambushed south of Ben Cat and suffered heavy loss, and was forced to withdraw to Command Post/8th Regiment at SubSector Ben Cat. 1/8th Battalion Command unit and 1st Company were ambushed and encircled at Bung Dia. Captain Cua and 1st Company fought back valiantly, and pushed back three enemy assaults, while giving order to 2nd Company in operation at Bung Cau to rush back to rescue the battalion. General Phong flew above the battlefield in order to direct in person the counterattack and resistance of 1/8th Battalion.

Troops' morale was high because of the division commander's presence; 2nd Company regrouped to attack enemy's rear from the south in order to pierce through the enemy's battalion command defensive line, forcing the enemy troops to scatter in panic. When General Phong landed his helicopter down to inspect enemy's casualties and captured weapons, he witnessed Captain Cua and the1st Company leader still holding grenades in their hands ready to fight to the end with the enemy. He recommended battlefield promotions to Captain Cua and the two company's leaders. The day he was promoted, Captain was saddened because the names of the two company's commanders were not listed on the promotion document. He consoled me by intervening with the division commander to let me attend the Class 7 of Battalion Commander in Dalat, in order to become the 1/9th Battalion Executive Officer to a new Battalion Commander, Captain Nguyen Van Vy, auguring a three year downfall phase in my military career.

When I received the transfer order to assume the 1/9th Battalion Executive Officer, Major Cua invited me to have dinner at his residence, in order to inquire the reason I ordered a Chinese civilian not to cater Vietnamese prostitutes to the American GIs at Lai Khe. I merely responded because it was a matter of national pride. He derided me because of my narrow mind and discriminatory attitude, and then he tried to investigate who had given me the order that was not in line with the TO&E (Table of Organization and Equipment). I was put in a dilemma, because of the two opposite directions taken by two of my superiors; nevertheless, I did not want Captain Vy to assume the responsibility of the order he had given me because I had promised before executing this out of TO&E mission; that was why I did not reveal the truth to Captain Cua, and accepted full consequence of my foolish action. Later on, I came to know that my new commander was also a competent general: he had infused new life to 5th Division by appointing many young officers of the VNMA into leadership positions, such as LTC Chau Minh Kien, an ARVN hero and an exceptional battalion commander of Class 19/VNMA, as 1/8th Battalion Commander, Captain Thieu of Class 19/VNMA as 4/8th Battalion Commander, Captain Nguyen Ky Suong as 2/8th Battalion Commander, Captain Le Sy Hung as 5th Recon Company Leader; furthermore, my new commander gallantly approved my transfer to VNMA as I wished in the beginning of 1969, and he also approved my advanced training in the United States prior to my VNMA's transfer. It was LTC Cua who made the recommendation to General Hieu to commute my transfer order to VNMA upon my return from abroad to assume the position of 1/8th Battalion Commander in the end of 1969.

Each time I visited him when he was Binh Duong Province Chief, he expressed concerns about the life and security of the population, which reminded me of Aspirant Lieutenant Bui Thuong, the heroic longrange scout some few years ago. Because of his love toward the population, he was kept at the province chief position for more than 5 years until the fall of the country, although he had requested to command a combat unit several times. In the beginning of April 1975, he reiterated to me on the international long distance telephone line that he would stay to fight with the combatants, and would not flee the country. He kept his promise and died in the communist prison, as a classmate of mine, Nguyen Van Hiep, told me.

BRIGADIER GENERAL TRAN THANH PHONG

When Captain Cua and the three Company's commanders just came out of Brigadier General Tran Thanh Phong's office, Captain Hoang, Class 15/VNMA, pulled me aside and whispered to me, "The Commander is understanding, don't you dare be insolent or troublesome!" I retorted, "Didn't you teach me to talk frankly!" He threw a condescending look at me, "OK, let me apologize to the Commander since I have taught you to behave that way." I don't know how Hoang had persuaded General Phong, but from that moment on I noticed that the General changed his leadership style entirely, from haughty to friendly, from commanding a battle from his office to shouldering the combatants on the battlefield fearlessly. It was unfortunate that he left the 5th Division too soon and did not get the chance to make use of his talents after his metamorphic change.

BRIGADIER GENERAL LE NGUYEN VY

Brigade General Le Nguyen Vy was the person who sympathized with my downfall when he was still 9th Regiment Commander. Whenever he visited the battalion, he did not fail to mention to me that my transfer from one battalion to another was beyond his authority.

Oftentimes, at lighter moment, he advised me to seek an audience with the "Authority" to present the truth because Captain Nguyen Van Vy, my former 1/8th Battalion Commander, had just left the army. Seeing that he could not convince me after three years, he counseled me go to the United States for further training and to request to be transferred to the VNMA where I would be of better service. Meanwhile, he assigned me to the regimental command unit to spend time playing chess with him and listening to his military career stories. The reason he joined the military was similar to Captain Cua's; however, he had a wider strategic vision than Captain Cua, in that he was concerned that the antiwar movements in the United States would strongly affect the American policy in the future; he tried to find a strategy of "SelfSufficiency" for the ARVN in case the Americans gave up Vietnam. The twomonth period living with him allowed me to know him to be a devoted patriot with a fanatic anti communist stance.

When I returned to my country, I learned the news that the order of my transfer to the VNMA had been canceled. I realized at this moment that my destiny was still attached to the 5th Infantry Division. When he met me, he told me the good news that the curse cast on me all these years had been dispelled by a visionary and charismatic leader, Major General Nguyen Van Hieu. While awaiting my assignment to 1/8th Battalion, I again listened to his passionate discourses on the topic of selfsufficiency although he had not found how to implement it.

Neither was he satisfied with my understanding of the antiwar movement in the United States, which made him decide to travel to the United States to get further training as a means to get a better understanding of this issue. A few days prior to my return to 1/8th Battalion, he proudly recounted the outstanding military exploits of 1/8th Battalion under the command of LTC Chau Minh Kien, Class 19/VNMA, then his sorrow when he witnessed the deterioration and defeat of the battalion in the Iron Triangle area after LTC Kien's death in action. He was also ashamed in finding out that the accomplishment of 1/8th Battalion was pale in comparison to an American battalion's in the Dong Tien program after the death of LTC Kien; he then told me this was the opportunity to know what it means by national disgrace if 1/8th Battalion performs worse than an ally unit.

One month later, he was elated in seeing that the achievements of 1/8th Battalion were 4 times more better than an ally battalion (see Assessment of 5th Infantry Division). He liked the most the "Insert, Move, Mine, Assault, Extract" tactic used in the Iron Triangle. Before saying goodbye to 1/8th Battalion, he was proud and happy like a kid when he witnessed the Platoon Leader of the Recon Platoon/1/8th Bn training his recon platoon and the American's in the use of this new tactic; in particular how to transform a manually controlled Claymore into an automatic mine, or an artillery shell into an automatic or a controlled mine.

In the beginning of 1974, he phoned to inquire about my well-being and to ask if I wanted to return to 5th Division or not. I honestly let him know that I had been ordered by General Tho to prepare myself to go to the United States for advanced training. In the middle of April 1974, he sent an emissary to An Dong Officers Club to tell me to come to see him before my departure to the United States. He was at that time a Colonel and a Division Commander. He appeared older and more majestic than four years before, but he was still enthusiastic and energetic as before. He asked why I had to go to training during the current critical situation of the country. I honestly presented to him that my new plan of action was to fight against the antiwar movement and the leftwing news media, and also my intention to submit my request for military discharge while I was studying abroad. He hastily took out a small notebook to transcribe names and addresses of a few students studying abroad and of Americans that he had tried to rally to his cause during the oneyear he was studying abroad and gave them to me. I asked his opinion about the Paris Agreement. He reiterated his predictions he formulated when he played chess with me in 1969, however he stated that he would fight to the end with his soldiers. Finally, he advised me to visit General Hieu before I went abroad. Sensing my hesitation to go to Bien Hoa, he told me to go outside to chat with Suong, Class 16/VNMA and wait for him. After about 15 minutes, he called me in and let me know that General Hieu would have lunch at noon in the An Dong Officers Club the following week and he wished to meet me there. I stood up and solemnly saluted a "Samurai" warrior of the 20th century.

MAJOR GENERAL LAM QUANG THO AND HIS GENERAL STAFF

A month of working at the Organization Bureau of the VNMA had made me aware of the complexities and difficulties of a general staff officer. In the past, VC sappers had infiltrated and attacked twice the VNMA, they even penetrated deeply and opened fire in the office of the VNMA commandant. Following two attacks, they assassinated the cadet military affairs director, an honest and model colonel, while he was asleep in his bedroom at the Cadets' Regiment. The new Table of Organization & Equipment (TO&E)

that my two predecessors, Organization Bureau Chiefs, had prepared, was still not approved by the JGS after several submissions… Nevertheless, that did not prevent me from performing smoothly my task of a general staff officer with Major General Lam Quang Tho until an incident occurred on the graduation day of Class 25 in the end of 1972. After that incident, I lived under constant pressure when I had to perform tasks that were not defined in the TO&E pertaining to an organization bureau chief assigned by General Tho, beyond the normal tasks of a general staff officer.

According to TO&E, the Organization Bureau was tasked to organize operations, to train cadets in general staff, to secure the defense of the facilities and to organize the graduation of the cadets. On the Graduation Day of Class 25/VNMA, General Cao Van Vien's attaché conveyed a wrong departure time to the General. Therefore, the General took his time eating breakfast, while General Tran Thien Khiem, the presiding VIP of the Graduation Ceremony, had departed on time as planned. When I discovered the gaff, there wasn't sufficient time to report it to General Tho, so I took it upon myself to give order to General Khiem's attaché to have the car stop at Ho Xuan Huong for sightseeing, then I gave order to General Vien's attaché to urge the General to skip his breakfast and to hurry up to arrive at the ceremony stand before General Khiem. General Tho was standing 10 meters nearby and saw troops of the Prime Minister's Security team pointing their weapons at me while I calmly gave out the order in the name of General Tho without seeking prior approval of General Tho. Today, I seize this opportunity to apologize to both of you, General Khiem and General Vien, and appreciate your magnanimity in not reprimanding me for causing inconvenience to both of you in the graduation ceremony of Class 25/VNMA in 1972. In particular General Vien had approved my promotion to the rank of Lieutenant Colonel and had selected me for attending advanced training in the United States in 1974. Despite the fact I did not act as dictated by general staff's principle, the ceremony was a success and General Tho submitted the request for my promotion to the rank of Lieutenant Colonel. He then went on instruct me to perform many other tasks that were out of line in terms of general staff's principle from that day until the day I went to the United States to attend my advanced training in 1974.

During the time I served a combat unit at company and battalion levels, I was not at all aware of the power held by MACV in Saigon; however, I came to know it when I assumed the task of preparing the draft of a new TO&E for VNMA. Just like my two predecessors at the helm of the Organization Bureau, the new TO&E draft was still rejected by the JGS two more times. Out of desperation I sought advice with General Tho who taught me the right way to proceed. I was told to bypass the military hierarchical ladder and to contact directly with MACV in Saigon. And that was it! The new TO&E was approved; general staff officers as well as other cadres would benefit from the same promotion criteria as those in combat units. General Tho valued the dedication of officers serving at the academy and was very pleased with this new TO&E because it allowed him to submit promotion requests for officers of the general staff, the instruction staff and cadres in the Cadets' Regiment.

To counter internal enemy cells, General Tho ordered me to devise a counterattack plan, totally different from the official defensive plan issued to commanders of key positions, to be submitted solely to him for review. He cautioned me that this secret plan should be known only to him and me, and told me, when circumstances required such as his absence during the enemy attack … I would execute this secret plan in his name. This out of line order panicked me and I made the suggestion to disseminate it also to the Chief of Staff to avoid my career being shortchanged as when I was with 1/8th Battalion. He revealed to me other incredible information about my Chief of Staff: he had been under military security's monitoring quite a long time; therefore he could not be entrusted with the lives of cadets. It made me more insecure having to work with a Chief of Staff under investigation; I asked General Tho why the military security didn't just catch him. He told me that this was how the professional counterintelligence people operated. Besides, this was the beauty of a free and democratic system, entirely different with the "Rather make mistakes in killing than overlook a target" policy of the Communists; they kill the persons they have suspicion while we only condemn somebody when we have evidences in our hands.

A few weeks later, he engaged me in another game that was not within the role of the Organization Bureau as defined by the TO&E. He instructed me to organize in secrecy the intelligence network involving the civilian population in the areas of Ap Thai Phien and Khu Chi Lang. I immediately tried to avoid performing that task under the pretext that I had never undergone training in intelligence; and I also respectfully made him know of my repulsion toward the spying game or the use of back door alleys. He simply rebutted me by saying, "Well, aren't we part of the Military Academy!"

I did not like at all bypassing my chief of staff in performing my job because I knew it would create friction between the two of us, which would then affect negatively my subordinates; for that reason, I did not use them in these out of line tasks. General Tho's ordering directly the General Administration Bureau/VNMA to submit a request only for my promotion after the Class 25's graduation was the starting point for the rocking waves between the chief of staff and me, because my CofStaff suspected that I had bypassed him in soliciting directly General Tho. Three months later, I was promoted ad hoc LTC in a normal yearly promotion, which increased my Cof Staff's suspicion. Auguring the crashes was the CofStaff's refusal to submit the special promotion request for two officers who headed two sections in my Bureau, and Meritorious Certificates after the graduation ceremony, while many officers who headed sections in other bureaus were awarded with Meritorious Certificates. The CofStaff took over my office, and moved my office around from one location to another about three or four times. He gave order to the Officer, Head of Defense and Security Section of the Organization Bureau, to accompany cadets on mission in Central Vietnam, despite the fact I had advised him that the Officer, Head of Defense and Security Section, did not have to go with the cadets and it did not correspond to his function as defined in the TO&E of the Organization Bureau a tactical operation officer and an instructor of general staff to cadets. The CofStaff created internal disturbance in the Organization Bureau by inciting the officer in charge of operations in the Tactical Operation Center to disobey my order. One night, I came to the TOC to inspect ambush positions of the LongRange Recon Squad. I was surprised to find out that one key ambush position to intercept the enemy's communication line at Thai Phien hamlet had been ordered by the CofStaff to be moved to another position, which was tactically unsound. I seized this opportunity to test the CofStaff by telling the officer in charge of operations to have the ambush team revert to its original position. He refused to obey my order, and called the CofStaff to report my order and awaited new order from the CofStaff. The CofStaff ordered him to execute my order. As for the security clearance issue of my CofStaff and the cadet safety matter, I determined it was about time to voice my disagreement to the CGS for only one issue, his infringement with general staff principle– the TOC was under direct control of the Organization Bureau– I disciplined the Officer in charge of operations with a 15-day internment for disobeying the immediatesuperior and for bypassing military hierarchical protocol, with the intention to test the CofStaff's reaction. He was clever in agreeing with me and in not interfering any more with the Organization Bureau; nevertheless, the relationship between the CofStaff and me became tense since that moment.

I started to get tired of this cat and mouse situation and resorted to study mathematics to ease off the tension of my mind. General Tho sympathized with my predicament and advised me to study journalism and he then would nominate me for training in the United States. I followed his advice and registered to take the second year of journalism at Van Hanh University in Saigon. A classmate of Class 17/VNMA helped me in getting course lessons from Saigon, and I was able to study and passed the course without difficulty. Early 1974, General Tho let me know that I was approved to attend the CGS in the United States. It was during that period that I came to know the personality and competence of General Tho. He complained about the deterioration in the quality of meals served to the cadets due to inflation, although he had set up a strict monitoring system of thefts. He felt confident in the area of defense because he just learned of the imminent military discharge of the CofStaff for reasons of personal security; and he had the civilian intelligence under control. He understood the need for psychological warfare against news media and the enemy's propaganda in the United States ... His convincing arguments had helped me in transforming from a rigid professional soldier to a flexible loner venturing in a far away country. In February 1975, General Tho sent me the news I would be honorably discharge from the army as my wish in order to pursue my new path in life.

After 1975, I learned that my CofStaff was a spy for COSVN, which made me admire more General Tho; and I stopped regretting performing those tasks not in line with general staff's principle while I served under such a competent general.

MAJOR GENERAL NGUYEN VAN HIEU

Major General Nguyen Van Hieu was the person who had provided me with the chance to getting out of my destitute condition during my period of downfall and for me into a period full of challenges and adventures which fulfilled the dream of a soldier. He had appointed me to my position without any personal gains and solely based on my military records and the recommendations of Colonels Nguyen Van Cua and Le Nguyen Vy. He had saved my life, without being aware of it, when he flew his C&C helicopter above my head in a rapid counterattack against a sapper squad of a VC battalion, which planned to attack the 5th Infantry Division HQ in Lai Khe in early 1970. He had demonstrated his sense of responsibility, courage, shrewdness and competence of a field commander defending the frontier, when he shouldered the combatants of 8th Task Force in the 1971 Snoul Operation. Furthermore, he was an honest and virtuous general, with a clear vision of the political and strategic behindthescenes in the national and international stages. He was indeed a visionary and charismatic leader of the Republic of Vietnam that Vietnam had lacked for more than a century; however, opportunity presented itself too late to allow him to deploy his talents. In late 1972, he had demonstrated to me his anticommunist patriotism and shared with me his predictions pertaining to the new policy adopted by the United States after the visit to Red China by Nixon.

Just one hour eating lunch with him at the An Dong Officers' Club in late April 1974, I knew he was an outstanding international strategist, besides his outstanding intellectual and military talents. He understood clearly the danger of losing the country after the Paris Agreement, the antiwar movement in the United States, the Watergate scandal of President Nixon and the law limiting the war power of the United States President. Nevertheless, he remained steadfast with policies of "Drinking to the Last

Drop", "Finishing the Job Despite Allies' Dropout", "Fighting Tooth and Nail Against the Enemy"... He had a ready plan for "Delaying Tactical War" with a diplomatic line of action in the international arena; however, "Man Proposes and God Disposes", and conditions did not allow him to save the match move against the Republic of Vietnam.

When I accompanied him to the parking lot, I came to realize that a new mission which was not in line with the TO&E was awaiting me when General Hieu revealed to me the letter President Nixon had sent to President Thieu in which he promised with Thieu the United States would intervene in the Vietnam War if the VC transgressed seriously the agreement. I respectfully saluted the visionary and charismatic leader, a "Samurai" warrior of the 20th Century.

In July 1975, I released a sounding balloon about the letter of promise although I failed to find a copy after almost living a year in the United States. However, my action got me an introduction letter from the White House to meet with the Delegate of VC Observer in the United Nations in New York. After a threehour presentation of General Hieu's will in a tiny room near the rooftop of a skyscraper, I went home with hope about the outcome final phase of the war. However I had failed when I learned that military and civilian cadres of South Vietnam continued to be imprisoned and when I learned about the mysterious death of Dinh Ba Thi, the person who had listened to my sincere presentation, I knew right away that Le Duan and the Communist Party had discarded the patriot will of General Hieu. Then the changing events in history had shown me the damaging consequences of the country when Le Duan rejected General Hieu's will: the VietnameseChinese War, the relinquishing of in land and sea land territories to Red China, the imbalance in the international strategy for Vietnam nowadays...

THOUGHTS OF AN ARVN SOLDIER

The Vietnam War has its origin way back in the 18th century, when Nguyen Anh sought help from the army of a foreign country in defeating a national hero, King Quang Trung.

Following were the waves of colonialism, of economical and cultural expansionism that European countries imposed on Asian underdeveloped countries, then the "Containment Doctrine" carried out by the United States in Southeast Asia. Challenged by these enormous pressures, some countries were able to withstand and preserve their independence and traditional culture such as Thailand, while Vietnam was devastated, colonized and destroyed. History shows that the foreign policy and the character of Thailand had helped avoid the strategic chess game of foreign powers, while the wrong foreign policy adopted by the Kings of the Nguyen Dynasty and the character of the Vietnamese had contributed in placing Vietnam on the orbits designed by chess players from foreign countries. This is an important topic for ethnologists in exploring the differences between the people from Thailand and from Vietnam, in order to facilitate the necessary transformation of the Vietnamese character in its attempt to end the ideologically civil Vietnam War, which is reaching its final stage.

I grew up and then became a soldier of the ARVN; and therefore I only write from the perspective of a tiny pawn on the international chessboard dominated by chess players of foreign countries. As a consequence of the sudden withdrawal of one of the chess players — The United States — the ARVN had failed in defending the people of the South who cherish freedom and democracy. Nevertheless, the ARVN was an army with a just cause and its own pride. The ARVN soldiers had a clear understanding of their role in the fight against the Communists in order to defend the freedom of South Vietnam. On the other hand, the Communist Party was successful in deceiving the NVA soldiers into fighting for atheist communism, which is against their own traditional beliefs and their own ways of life. The ARVN soldiers like the government of the RVN had no other choice in receiving allies' aid, but they categorically refused to become any foreign countries' slaves. The North Vietnamese Communists, on the contrary, while also forced to seek aid from the Communist Bloc, agreed to become its slaves, like in the cases of land reform in the North, of 1975 invasion of the South under Russian pressure...The ARVN was also unfortunate in the lack of national leadership, while the North Communists got a cunning and cruel leader, Ho Chi Minh, and hid their undertaking under the label of fighting against the French and then the Americans to defend the country. The ARVN and the RVN government demonstrated humanitarian concern in carrying out a bloodless land reform, as well as magnanimity toward the Communists in implementing the openarm and humanitarian prisoner policy, while the Communists treated with cruelty and without consideration of human rights the South Vietnamese combatants when they agreed to lay down their weapons in order to avoid an unnecessary bloodshed in a fight that had reached its final stage. History's timeline has shown that the North Vietnamese Communists committed widespread missteps: the secret agreement with the Chinese Communists of ceding in land and sea land territories, the corruption and discord amidst Communist rank and file, and the poverty and the chaos in the Vietnam society. It also has shown the shameful transgression of the North Vietnamese Communists before the scrutiny of the opinion and the history of the Vietnam War. Today, the despicable conduct of a few overseas Vietnamese when they returned to their country, the overzealous anticommunist outburst of a few Vietnamese residents abroad, the machiavellian machinations of some individuals, or the subservient bargaining with foreign superpowers, all these are consequences of the wrong, mischievous and petty policy of the North Vietnamese Communists.

A conflict can only be resolved peacefully and permanently with both sides jointly building up the country when they have mutual respect and mutual compassion. The North Vietnamese Communists are having the upper hand at the present time. Therefore it's their responsibility to put an end the ideologically civil conflict—democracy and communism.

This requires that they have the courage and patriotism to put away their current unstable and legally unfounded powers. Such is the condition of Vietnam, which wants to escape the dominance of the two foreign chess players who are now commencing a new game in our beloved Vietnam. Let's wait and see!

Tran Van Thuong 19 June 2006
generalhieu.com